Healing Hormones

How to Turn On Natural Chemicals to Reduce Stress

Mark J. Estren, Ph.D.
Beverly A. Potter, Ph.D.

RONIN
Berkeley CA

Healing Hormones

How to Turn On
Natural Chemicals
to Reduce Stress

Mark J. Estren, Ph.D.
Beverly A. Potter, Ph.D.

Healing Hormones

Copyright 2013: Mark J. Estren & Beverly A. Potter
ISBN: 978-1-57951-167-8

Published by
Ronin Publishing, Inc.
PO Box 22900
Oakland, CA 94609
www.roninpub.com

Production:
Cover & Book Design: Beverly A. Potter
Editor: Mark J. Estren

Library of Congress Card Number: 2013951046
Distributed to the book trade by PGW/Perseus

Orandum est ut sit mens sana in corpore sano.
Fortem posce animum mortis terrore carentem,qui
spatium vitae extremum inter munera ponat naturae.

—Juvenal, 2nd century C.E.

You should pray for a healthy mind in a healthy
body. Ask for a strong heart that has no fear of death,
and deems the length of your life the least of Nature's gifts.

Other Books by Dr. Mark J. Estren

A History of Underground Comics
Statins: Miraculous or Misguided?
Prescription Drug Abuse

Table of Contents

Introduction

THE JOB INTERVIEW is going to be stressful. Mary really needs the work. She knows she's qualified, but she knows that a hundred other people, maybe more, will be interviewing for the same position. She can't control her nervousness—her palms are sweaty and she won't even be able to give a firm handshake. She worries that she'll mess up in the first seconds of the interview. But fortunately, Mary knows about the power of healing hormones, so she came prepared. She reaches into her purse for a nasal spray. Within minutes after using it, Mary feels calmer and fully ready to face the interviewer. She radiates confidence and gets the job.

John and Ellen are both nervous about their first date. Ridiculous meeting like this—phony, artificial… set up by friends, but do friends really know what they are looking for? John and Ellen have the same thoughts and the same worries—but neither has any intention of revealing them to the other. We'll just sit, have dinner, talk a little and split, thinks John. That will be more than enough, thinks Ellen; never again! I really need to calm down, they both think at almost the same moment—unknowingly. And then both reach for small

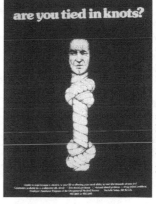

bottles of a hormonal nasal spray. Half an hour later, both are much more relaxed, open and receptive to new experience, wondering what they were so worried about a short while earlier. The date is a success and lasts for hours, and a second one soon follows.

Peter has Asperger's syndrome—an autistic spectrum disorder affecting a person's ability to socialize and communicate effectively with others. So Peter is socially very awkward; his behavior patterns are repetitive; he is physically clumsy and often uses the wrong word when nervous—as he often is. Doctors have told him there is nothing wrong with his intelligence—or, for that matter, his linguistic abilities. He just cannot bring them into play in appropriate ways—he cannot figure out the emotional content of what is said to him, and therefore gets muddled when he responds. At one appointment, Dr. Smithson suggests a hormone injection that may make things easier for Peter. *What do I have to lose?* Peter thinks. Dr. Smithson gives him the shot. Later that day, when talking to his sister, Peter feels as if a bright light has gone on in his brain: he understands what she is saying and the emotions behind it. He has a clear, straightforward talk with her—a small thing in most people's lives, but a huge one in Peter's.

> *You can heal yourself through your body's own everyday functions.*

Healing Hormones

WOULDN'T IT BE NICE if all life's little problems, and some of its big ones, could be handled this easily? These stories are exaggerations, but not by much. They build on solid scientific research on the effect of capturing mood-altering or mood-enhancing substances called hormones that our bodies manufacture naturally, and using specific hormones as supplements to make our lives better.

In this book, you will learn about five healing hormones that have specific positive functions in the body—helping you relax, function better, even have a stronger heart and cardiovascular system. And you will learn how you can have more of these natural substances in your body—in some cases through a nasal spray like the ones Mary, John and Ellen used, in others through an injection like the one Dr. Smithson gave Peter, and in still others simply by making more of the healing hormones yourself.

That's right. Intriguingly, scientists have found that there are ways of harnessing our bodies' own abilities to make healing hormones—which means you can learn how to help yourself, heal yourself, through your body's own everyday functions.

What Hormones Are

WHAT EXACTLY ARE healing hormones? A hormone is simply a chemical released by a cell, a gland, or an organ in one part of the body that affects cells in other parts of the body. Hormones are chemical messengers—transmitters—that transport some sort of signal from one cell to another. *Healing* hormones transport signals that make us feel better—calmer, more relaxed, better able to cope with everyday life. They are among the hormones produced by one specific organ: the brain. And what they do is transmit nerve impulses to other nerves, muscles or glands. Healing hormones are there-fore in a group called *neurotransmitters*, with "neuro-" meaning "nerve." But the word does not refer to one specific nerve—it relates to the entire *nervous system*, the vast network of nerve cells and fibers that transmits nerve impulses among parts of the body. A slight increase in a healing hormone has significant whole-body effects that you can learn to produce on your own.

The stories of Mary, John, Ellen and Peter all show the effects of one particular healing hormone, *oxytocin*, which is released into the bloodstream when people experience love, closeness and cuddling. As we shall see, the effects of oxytocin are more wide-ranging than they were once thought to be: oxytocin works in some rather complex ways to cement all sorts of human connections—and can treat some conditions that have previously been considered unmanageable.

Healing Neurotransmitters

OXYTOCIN IS one of the neurotransmitters that function as healing hormones. "Neurotransmitter" is a scientific term; "healing hormone" is a simple way to think of what these chemicals do in and for your body. Another healing hormone is dopamine, which produces feelings of pleasure and motivation, and can be used to alleviate some severe conditions, including clinical depression and Parkinson's disease. Still another healing hormone, nitric oxide, causes blood vessels to dilate—that is, to enlarge—which protects against cardiovascular disease, helping prevent stroke and heart attack. Then there are endorphins, healing hormones that fight stress and relieve pain. And there is serotonin, which can be thought of as a happiness hormone, boosting relaxation and overall good bodily feelings, and promoting sound sleep.

Neurotransmitters have distinct effects on the body, some pleasant and others that are not pleasant at all.

By describing specific neurotransmitters as healing hormones, we are deliberately placing a value judgment on chemicals that do certain things rather than others. But the healing hormones are only a few members of the large class of neurotransmitters. The first neurotransmitter discovered, *acetylcholine*, was identified by German pharmacologist Otto Loewi in 1921—in an experiment with two frog hearts that came to

> *The body's chemicals are not at war with each other, but it certainly feels that way at times.*

him in a dream. Loewi was awarded the Nobel Prize in Physiology or Medicine in 1936 for his work, which proved acetylcholine to be a chemical substance carrying signals across synapses in the brain. This discovery revealed that most communication between nerve cells and other cells is not electrical, as many had believed, but chemical.

Since Loewi's discovery, many other neurotransmitters have been found, and most people are familiar with some of them even without knowing that they *are* neurotransmitters. The reason for the familiarity is that these chemicals have distinct effects on the body—some of them pleasant and to be encouraged, including the effects of the healing hormones, but others that are not pleasant at all. Understanding the healing hormones and learning to use them starts with an understanding of the neurotransmitters whose effects are *countered* by the healing hormones. You can think of the healing hormones and certain other neurotransmitters as antagonists in an ongoing battle for supremacy. In reality, the body's chemicals are not at war with each other, but it certainly feels that way at times.

In *Healing Hormones*, you will learn important truths about how your body functions, how it responds to everyday events instantaneously and without your conscious control, and how you can take advantage of substances that your body makes on its own to live a calmer, less-frenetic, less-stressed life. In fact, stress— what it is, what causes it, what it represents, and what the healing hormones can help you do about it—is a good place to start.

1:

Stressors

WE USE THE WORD "stress" loosely in everyday life: "I'm so stressed." "That meeting was so stressful." "I got stuck in traffic—what stress!" "Stop stressing me—I'll get to it as soon as I can." But what exactly *is* stress? All these colloquial uses share an underlying error: they treat stress as something that *happens to us*. Not so. Stress is a *response* to a situation—specifically a response to *change*.

Change is the most ubiquitous stressor—a stressor simply being anything that causes stress. Any change, even change for the better, is stressful. Change requires adjusting to new conditions, and is threatening because it brings uncertainty and possible loss of control. Loss of control and feeling helpless in the face of events are stressors. When you cannot control situations, circumstances could turn against you.

Stress is a necessary element of life: the right amount of it, not too little and not too much, is adaptive, helping us cope with the inevitable changes in our external environment. Change inevitably triggers stress, whether the change is for better or worse. The issue for most of us is that we live in the midst of so many changes that we practically always feel a degree of stress—and that is bad for our health.

Stress and Change

THE STRESS-CHANGE RELATIONSHIP has been well-known since at least 1967, when psychiatrists Thomas Holmes and Richard Rahe created the *Holmes and Rahe Stress Scale*—a list of 43 life events that they used to determine the relationship between life events and the likelihood of illness. Holmes and Rahe called their listing the "Social Readjustment Rating Scale" and used it to predict the likelihood of people becoming physically ill when certain events occurred in their lives. Holmes and Rahe assigned each life event a number of "life change units," ranging from 11 to 100, and had people self-report the number of events that had happened in their lives in the past year. Then they totaled the units—and found that certain totals really did predict physical illness.

> *Change, any change—negative or positive—can trigger the stress response*

Response to Instability

THE IMPORTANT THING to understand about the Holmes and Rahe scale, from the standpoint of healing hormones, is that the events on the scale are not necessarily negative. Thus, the stress produced by the events is a response to significant changes in one's life, even when those changes are pleasant ones. The Holmes and Rahe scale reveals that change—even positive change, such as getting married, having a child, or getting a new job—produces stress. Stress is thus a response to something out of the ordinary, which in the dim past would generally have been something negative—attack by a wild animal, for example—but which nowadays may be a positive event that knocks us out of the stable groove in which we generally live day to day.

Under the Holmes and Rahe scale, a total score of 300 or above puts a person at risk of illness; the risk is moderate—30% lower—for scores of 150 to 299; and the risk is only slight for scores below 150. The highest number of life change units is assigned to the death of a spouse: 100. Here are other examples, positive as well as negative.

Holmes-Rahe Scores

Divorce	73
Marital separation	65
Imprisonment	63
Death of close family member	63
Personal injury or illness	53
Marriage	50
Marital reconciliation	45
Change in financial state	38
Change in work responsibilities	29
Outstanding personal achievement	28
Vacation	13
Christmas	12

You have probably heard that stress is associated with something called the "fight or flight response." Walter Bradford Cannon, M.D., coined the phrase "fight or flight" in 1915, and created a theory that is now widely accepted: we react to threats through the sympathetic nervous system, whose release of chemicals happens without our conscious control and gets us ready to fight a threat or get away from it. So a stressor, biologically speaking, is a stimulus that brings the sympathetic nervous system to full alert. This system normally percolates

> Today's threats are more likely to be emotional than physical.

along below our awareness, helping keep the body in *homeostasis*, which means in a stable, relatively constant condition. In effect, the body is in a "comfort zone" where all is well. And then, when something changes— that is, when a positive or negative stressor appears— the sympathetic nervous systems revs up very quickly.

Emergency Response

THINK OF the sympathetic nervous system as the body's emergency-response system. When something destabilizes the body's homeostasis, the sympathetic nervous system uses the body's energy to raise blood pressure, speed up heartbeat, and slow down digestion. To get its messages out to the body, the sympathetic nervous system uses hormones—neurotransmitters that are in the same class as healing hormones but that have a very different effect and are sometimes thought of as being in combat with healing hormones, since they do more-or-less opposite things.

The primary fight-or-flight hormones are *cortisol*, *epinephrine*, also called *adrenaline*, and *norepinephrine*. These hormones cause the body to behave in ways that are characteristic of the fight-or-flight effect: in addition to changes in blood pressure, heart rate and digestive processes, the pupil of the eye dilates—enlarges— to allow more light in, making it easier to see what to do and where to go; the bronchioles, which carry air to the lungs, also dilate, so more air is available in case a burst of speed for escape or attack is necessary; and there are effects on the sweat glands, kidneys and other organs as well.

Today's threats, however, tend to be emotional or psychological—worries about debt, for instance—rather than the physical threat of being eaten by a tiger. The body does not distinguish between the two forms of threat: both types trigger release of stress hormones. The entire sympathetic nervous system is built for fast, short bursts of stress hormones to mobilize us to leap out of the way of a tiger—or, for that matter, a speeding car. However, when threats are emotional and ongoing, without any quick physical resolution possible, we can find ourselves feeling unrelenting stress that can pose a hazard to our health. The reason for this is that the stress response is all or nothing: when a destabilizing threat is detected, the body responds—stress hormones ramp up specific bodily functions whether the perceived danger is physical or not. And this is why the fight-or-flight response has become such a negative element in so many people's lives.

So it is in this context that we can think about cortisol, a major stress hormone whose effects on the body—increasing blood sugar, suppressing the immune system, and aiding in the metabolism of fat, protein and carbohydrates—are well known and have long been studied. When mobilization for fight-or-flight is constant, cortisol levels remain elevated over the long term, which is more than the body was built to handle. Under these circumstances, cells in the immune system break

> *The stress response is all or nothing.*

down, promoting the development of autoimmune diseases as well as increasing vulnerability to other illnesses and making it harder for the body to fight off future infections. This is exactly what Holmes and Rahe were getting at when studying life-changing events and assigning each of them a score in units. The psychiatrists were looking for ways to identify which people under psychological stress were most likely to become physically ill. Thanks to the Holmes and Rahe scale, healthcare workers focusing on stress management know to look at three things:

Illness Precursors

A high frequency of major life-changing events affecting someone in the past year, such as divorce, death in the family, or a change in job, in accordance with the Holmes and Rahe scale.

The person's subjective perception that daily demands exceed his or her coping resources and/ or support system.

The person's current emotional state—feeling overwhelmed by life events.

So the question is: what can you do to reduce your likelihood of developing illnesses that are associated with the stressors—that is, perceived threats to homeostasis—of everyday life? The first "pointer," the one based on the Holmes and Rahe scale, is one over which you have little, if any, control: a death in the family or the loss of a job can happen anytime, and other Holmes and Rahe life events—such as sexual difficulties, taking on a mortgage or a change in social activities—will bring stress-related "units" with them and can be difficult to modify.

Our bodies have a wonderful array of self-correcting and self-balancing mechanisms, intended to keep us in homeostasis when threats are occasional and overcome quickly through the fight-or-flight response. Unfortunately, the constant stream of threats to which we are subjected in modern

> Psychological stress may set the stage for diseases associated with a weakened immune system.

life—usually non-physical ones that the body reacts to *as if* they are physical—makes it difficult for the self-correction mechanism to function optimally. This is where you and your ability to manufacture healing hormones come in. The basic question is: if cortisol, adrenaline/epinephrine and norepinephrine are stress hormones produced in response to signals from the sympathetic nervous system, are there "de-stress" hormones that turn them off or neutralize them, perhaps produced by some other bodily system? And the answer is yes: that is exactly what healing hormones do.

2:

Effects of Stressors

BEFORE CONSIDERING WAYS to reduce the stress response and thus make it easier for your body to produce more healing hormones, it is useful to examine in more detail the effects that a constant feeling of being stressed has on you. Physiologically, the stress response is essentially an overload of the hormones *cortisol*, *epinephrine* or *adrenaline*, and *norepinephrine*, which, like the healing hormones, are neurotransmitters with specific and significant functions in the body. It is important not to demonize these self-produced chemicals, which are crucial for many bodily processes. Epinephrine, for example, regulates heart rate and the diameter of blood vessels and air passages. And it is crucial for the fight-or-flight response, without which the human race might not have made it to its current lofty—if that is the right word—status.

But an oversupply of stress hormones produces a series of symptoms with which, unfortunately, most of us are all too familiar. The phrase "anxiety attack" is well known, and so is the phrase "panic attack," which is essentially a more-intense version of anxiety attack. Both involve an overwhelming sense of impending danger or doom; fear of loss of control or even of death; and physical symptoms that include

> *An oversupply of stress hormones produces a series of symptoms with which, unfortunately, most people are all too familiar.*

accelerated heart rate, sweating, trembling, chills and hot flashes— sometimes in alternation, sometimes occurring together—as well as nausea and abdominal cramps, chest pain, headache, faintness and/or dizziness, hyperventilation and shortness of breath.

> Even without causing a full-blown anxiety or panic attack, the stress response takes a significant toll on the body.

Drawing the line between an intense anxiety attack and a panic attack is not easy and not really necessary—what is important is to realize that both are responses to the body's over-production of fight-or-flight hormones at a time when the original purpose of those hormones, to facilitate physical fighting or physical flight, is no longer applicable.

Stress-Hormone Cycle

LIKE HEALING HORMONES, stress hormones can become enmeshed in a cycle that causes them to increase and increase again. Anxiety and panic attacks, for example, can cause so much fear of another such attack that they can cause stress hormones to rise and thus *bring on* the very attack you fear. These attacks can have deep roots that make them very difficult to prevent: there appears to be a genetic component to them, and significant trauma in childhood, such as physical or sexual assault, can make a person more likely to experience them.

On the other hand, specific stress-provoking events can bring on anxiety and panic attacks no matter what your background has been, as the Holmes-Rahe scale indicates. The death or serious illness of a loved one, a major positive or negative change in your life—such as the birth of a child—or any sort of adult trauma can cause severe anxiety or even panic. And such an attack, especially if repeated, can lead to avoidance of social situations, depression, and increased risk of suicide or suicidal thoughts. These are precisely the symptoms that healing hormones counteract.

Even without causing a full-blown anxiety or panic attack, the stress response takes a significant toll on the body. What brings on the near-instantaneous bodily changes that occur in the fight-or-flight response are hormonal secretions from the *hypothalamus*, a gland at the base of the brain. The hypothalamus signals two structures to respond to a perceived threat: the *adrenal medulla* then secretes *epinephrine* or *adrenaline*, plus *norepinephrine*; and the *pituitary gland* secretes *adrenocorticotropic hormone* or ACTH—which in turn stimulates the adrenal glands to produce *cortisol*, a hormone that increases blood sugar, suppresses the immune system, and aids in the metabolism of fat, protein and carbohydrates.

This system operates on two levels simultaneously. On the "instant" level, the adrenaline arouses the sympathetic nervous system and reduces activity in the parasympathetic nervous system, a complementary portion of the body's functionality that tends to enforce a state of homeostasis. It is adrenaline that decreases digestion and increases sweating, pulse rate and blood pressure. It is norepinephrine that boosts heart rate and the brain's oxygen supply, initially triggers glucose release from energy stores, and increases blood flow to skeletal muscle. It is cortisol that enables the body to maintain steady supplies of blood sugar—necessary for longer-term handling of stress—through the ongoing release of glucose from the liver; cortisol also helps control swelling after an injury.

Immune Suppression

BUT CORTISOL ALSO SUPPRESSES the immune system—a function that can become a serious risk to health. The immune system is initially stimulated by a perceived threat, and this makes sense: the body may be injured and, if it is, will need greater immunity to handle survival and repair. Cortisol's role is to make sure that the heightened immune response does not go on for too long—not for more than a few minutes—by suppressing the immune system's stimulation and allowing the body to return to normal immune-system levels.

And this works well *unless a stress response continues to be present.* In that situation—which is often the case in modern life, where threats are not usually in the simple form of fleeing an attacking predator—cortisol's dampening effect on the immune system can create serious problems, up to and including shrinking of the thymus gland, one of the key immune tissues of the body.

In the human fight-or flight-response in prehistoric times, "fight" was manifested in aggressive, combative behavior; "flight" was manifested by fleeing potentially threatening situations, such as being confronted by a predator. Things are more complicated now, and fight-or-flight responses include a wider range of behaviors. For example, the fight response may show in angry, argumentative behavior, and the flight response may be manifested through social withdrawal or substance abuse. There are gender differences as well: men are generally more likely to respond to an emergency with aggression, a "fight" response, while women are generally more likely to turn to others for help, or attempt to defuse the situation—that is, to try to escape, which is a "flight" response.

Our bodies quickly judge situations to decide if they are threatening.

Our bodies very quickly judge a situation to decide whether or not it is threatening, based on both physical and psychological factors. This does not mean "judging" as in making an intellectual decision—it means our bodies respond to the perceived threat level, the potential for destabilization, and respond accordingly without our conscious intention or control.

Situations are commonly called "stressful," but this is loose language: stress is the *response* to a situation that removes the body from a state of homeostasis. It is actually easy to see that the situation itself is not the source of stress, since we all know people who respond very differently to identical situations. For example, someone with an intense fear of snakes will experience stress and a fight-or-flight response upon seeing a snake in the path, while someone experienced with the reptiles, such as a herpetologist, is more likely simply to observe the snake with interest and possibly even pick it up. Same circumstances, different reactions—one resulting in stress, one not.

Today's Threats

THE THREATS THAT TRIGGER fight-or-flight are quite different from those that were present when the response first evolved, as Holmes and Rahe realized. In primitive times, the threats were tigers hiding in the bush and other dangerous situations that could lead to being killed—and eaten. In modern life, we no longer fear running into tigers, but we now face the more-abstract threats that Holmes and Rahe enumerated, from job loss to debt or marital discord; and we also face destabilizing situations that are clearly positive but that nevertheless provoke feelings of being stressed, such as moving to a new home or starting a new, better job.

Our bodies, though, do not differentiate between the physical threats more common in the distant past and the threats of modern times, which are so often psychological and emotional. A threat is a threat, and the fight-or-flight response is triggered to deal with or flee from it. And there we are, mobilized by the sympathetic nervous system with increased heart rate; lung dilation, causing increased and rapid breathing; increased perspiration; decrease in digestive activity; and glucose release from the liver, to provide energy for combat or running away as fast as possible.

But where is there to run *to*? In primitive times, our bodies mobilized to fight or flee the tiger—and then go back to the balance of homeostasis. Today, the perceived threats are not only vague but also continuous. When threatened by fears of job loss and debt piling up, our bodies inevitably respond with the fight-or-flight response. But there is no way either to defeat or to flee from these modern threats. So we remain in the threatening situations continuously, which means that our

> *The sympathetic nervous system's response is the same whether a threat is physical or psychological.*

body stays in a state of readiness for long periods of time. This is a problem, because the body is not built to sustain continuous readiness—it wears us down, leading to imbalance, physical dysfunction, and disease, just as Holmes and Rahe discovered.

"Bad" Hormones?

ADRENALINE/EPINEPHRINE, norepinephrine and
cortisol are all hormones and are all neurotransmitters,
just like the healing hormones. They are sometimes
thought of as "bad," since they are integral to the stress
response to perceived threat and it is generally ac-
knowledged that, to put it colloquially, there

S*tress is a response.* is "too much stress" in modern life. But stress
is a *response.* So the real issue is that *you are
responding with a high level of stress to perceived
threats.* Remember that stress is a *reaction:* again, consider the example of two people responding differently
to a snake in the path, with one feeling stress and the
other staying completely calm.

Thus, adrenaline/epinephrine, norepinephrine and
cortisol are not "bad," because they perform necessary, even critical functions on an ongoing basis and,
in particular, when our bodies need to respond to *real,
external* threats. Today's human beings would not exist if
yesterday's had not had these neurotransmitters en-
abling the fight-or-flight response that made it possible
for *Homo sapiens* to thrive among creatures with more
speed, better-protected skin, better hunting instincts
and far more dangerous teeth and claws than humans
possessed.

Today, though, when we live amid near-constant
stressors in situations to which physical fight-or-flight
is an inadequate or unavailable response, the overproduction of stress hormones results in a speeded-up heart
rate or heart palpitations, general irritability, sleep problems, hypertension, increased appetite that frequently
leads to overeating, and sexual effects—such as diminished sex drive in men and irregular menstrual periods

in women. There are even specific diseases associated with heightened stress hormones, such as *Cushing's syndrome*, in which hypertension, depression and sexual dysfunction are accompanied by overwhelming fatigue, abdominal stretch marks, diabetes, and—primarily in women—growth of facial hair.

Disturbing Effects

MOST PEOPLE, thankfully, never get to the stage of Cushing's syndrome or full-blown panic attacks. But even the lesser effects of the stress response can be disturbing and even debilitating. A common one is the feeling that you just cannot think straight—and this is not your imagination. An overload of cortisol in the brain is a form of imbalance of hormone production: the adrenal gland, which makes both cortisol and epinephrine, also makes the anti-inflammatory steroid *dehydroepiandrosterone* or DHEA—and when the balance of these hormones is off, particularly on an ongoing basis, you feel worn out and overwhelmed, too exhausted to pull coherent thoughts together. Many other symptoms result from overproduction of fight-or-flight hormones, too: excessive weight gain, especially around the midsection; fragile or thin-seeming skin that bruises easily; and such personality changes as mood swings, generalized irritability, paranoia and more.

These negative effects of overproduction of stress hormones "take over" the body. One of the problems with many well-meaning suggestions about handling stressors is that they require you to get control of the stress response be-

> *Even the lesser effects of the stress response can be disturbing and even debilitating.*

fore you can take advantage of them—which is impossible. "Just do some yoga," for example, means "just get into a state of mind in which you can do yoga." But if you could get into that state of mind, you would not be so stressed! For some people, this is why the relaxation response (see next chapter) is not a good option: they cannot get themselves into a state of mind and body in which they can take advantage of it.

Nevertheless, there *are* ways to handle the stress response and the hormones that result from and reinforce it—and effective stress management, all by itself, goes a long way toward helping the body produce more healing hormones that will then, in a positive feedback loop, reduce the fight-or-flight reaction still further.

3:

Relaxation Response

TRY TO STAND and sit at the same time. Impossible! And it is just as impossible to be tense and relaxed at the same time. Prolonged tension is bad. It tightens us literally—we have all experienced muscular tightening and an overall "sprung-steel" feeling when tense. And it tightens us figuratively—making it hard to think clearly and engage our brains, energy and emotions. Extended periods of tension relate to ongoing activation of the body's *sympathetic nervous system,* which produces the fight-or-flight response through release of the hormones cortisol, epinephrine and norepinephrine. But this whole system was designed for short, intense bursts of activity, not prolonged periods of heightened awareness and arousal. When we remain in the grip of this system for a lengthy time, our hormones are essentially short-circuiting us, and even compromising our immune system—so that we become increasingly vulnerable to illness.

> We cannot be both tense and relaxed at the same time.

Just as you cannot sit and stand at the same time—just as the weather cannot get hotter and colder at the same time—certain things are incompatible with each other. And there is a psychological principle called *differential reinforcement of incompatible behavior* (DRI)

> *Deep relaxation brings on profound physiological changes including decreased metabolism, decreased blood pressure, slower heart rate, slowed rate of breathing, and more-relaxed brainwave patterns.*

that you can use to get more of what you want and less of what you do not want. Don't let the jargon distract you. All it means is that if two behaviors are incompatible, we can reinforce (strengthen) the one we want, which will automatically decrease (weaken) the one we do not want. So if we know that we cannot be tense and relaxed at the same time, and what we want is to be relaxed rather than tense, then by reinforcing (strengthening) our relaxation, we automatically decrease (weaken) our tension. We cannot have both at the same time. This is a principle underlying the relaxation response—a specific method of increasing our feelings of being relaxed and therefore, by definition, decreasing our feelings of tension.

Named in the 1960s at Harvard University by Herbert Benson, M.D., the relaxation response brings our bodies' *parasympathetic nervous system* into play to counter the effects of the *sympathetic nervous system*, which elicits the fight-or-flight response. If the sympathetic nervous system is thought of as stimulating, then the parasympathetic nervous system can be thought of as calming—and the two normally work together to keep the body balanced in homeostasis.

Dr. Benson discovered that when people practice deep relaxation, they undergo a set of profound physiological changes that are opposite to the ones caused by stress—including decreased metabolism, decreased blood pressure, slower heart rate, slowed rate of breathing, and more-relaxed brainwave patterns.

Why Relax?

OUR BODY DOES NOT MAKE a value judgment between the sympathetic and parasympathetic nervous
systems—both respond to external factors automatically, beneath our conscious control. But our conscious
mind *does* distinguish between tension and relaxation,
and at a conscious level most of us would generally prefer to be relaxed. Relaxation is a calm feeling. We feel
at peace with our environment. We consider ourselves
better able to cope with whatever is going on around us.
We think more clearly. We find solutions to problems.
We interact more warmly and pleasantly with those
around us. We sleep better and awake feeling more
refreshed. We consider ourselves to be in better control
of our thoughts and feelings. We can handle our environment better.

These positive feelings are
the result of our body's increasing
production of healing hormones—
and the physical results of that
production, as noted above, are
substantial. Our heart rate slows.

> *The relaxation
> response
> counteracts
> physical and
> emotional stress.*

Our breathing is slower and deeper.
Our blood pressure is lower. Our thinking is clearer. We
simply feel better. These are good things for our conscious mind and aware body.

How to Relax

THE FASTEST AND EASIEST WAY to elicit the relaxation response is by breathing deeply. To help you
experience this for yourself, we can first explore what
happens when we breathe rapidly.

Try this now.

Rapid Breathing

Using a scale of 1 to 10, rate how tense or relaxed
you feel right now—with extremely tense being 10
and very relaxed being 1. Now breathe quickly for
a minute. Stop and notice how you feel—and rate
yourself again on the same scale of 1 to 10.

If you are like most of us, you probably noticed that
your tension went up a little—maybe even a lot—when
you breathed rapidly. Fast, shallow breathing is the
kind of breathing we do naturally when frightened. It's
part of the fight-or-flight response, helping us to take
in extra oxygen needed for the extraordinary effort of
fighting or fleeing. Even though nothing was actually
threatening you, when you breathed rapidly your body
began acting as it does when you encounter an actual
threat. You may have felt your heart racing, for example. The reason is that your breathing activated the
sympathetic nervous system, which produced the effects
that it would normally create in response to a perceived
threat. It is something of an all-or-nothing response
that clicks in.

Now try this.

Breathing Slowly & Deeply

Before starting, again rate your level of tension on
a scale of 1 to 10, with 1 being very relaxed and 10
being extremely tense.

Now breathe in very slowly, all the way down to
your diaphragm, which should rise as your lungs

fill. Silently count "one" as you slowly breathe in deeply. Then pause and hold in the air in your lungs as you think "and." Notice how the fullness feels tight. Now count "two" as you slowly exhale the air. Keep exhaling even when your lungs feel empty, and notice the feeling of relaxation in your chest. Continue to hold your lungs empty for a moment or two as you think "and."

Repeat, breathing in and out slowly and deeply, while counting "one" as you breathe in deeply; then think "and" as you pause and hold your lungs empty for a moment. Then count "two" as you slowly exhale and think "and" as you pause to hold your lungs empty for a moment. Continue breathing in and out slowly and deeply for a minute or so as you count "one - and - two - and - one - and -two" repetitively and rhythmically.

Again, rate your level of tension on the same scale of 1 to 10, with 10 being extremely tense and 1 being very relaxed. How do you feel after breathing slowly and deeply for a minute? How does this compare to your tension level before breathing deeply?

Fast, shallow breathing engages the sympathetic nervous system. Slow, deep breathing does the opposite—it turns on the parasympathetic nervous system. Like sitting and standing, these are incompatible responses—it is not possible to have both systems operating at the same time. The parasympathetic nervous system counters the stress response with the relaxation response.

If you did not get the slowdown effect when the parasympathetic nervous system kicked in, try deep breathing again—for a little longer this time. The extra time may be needed to get the parasympathetic nervous system into full function. The reason for this is that the sympathetic nervous system ramps up very quickly so you can fight a threat or get away from it. The calming effect of the parasympathetic nervous system takes longer to take effect—it goes fully into effect only when there is enough time to be sure you are safe and there are no immediate threats in the vicinity.

Physiologically speaking, the relaxation response transforms many of the body's physical and emotional responses to stress into their opposites—decreased heart rate, lower blood pressure, slower and deeper breathing, and less muscle tension. And it connects directly to the body's production of healing hormones. You can easily learn to produce a simple version of the relaxation response, which you can use when you are feeling stressed to lower that stress-related feeling that your body is "spinning out of control."

Monkey Mind

MUCH OF OUR THINKING TRIGGERS the stress response. Most of us have many stressors in our lives. Just thinking about them triggers the stress response. We worry about our kids, our relationships, our finances, our future, our health—on and on and on. We can "drive ourselves crazy" with our thinking. Buddhists, who have developed methods for quieting the mind, call this relentless chatter

> Much of our thinking triggers the stress response.

"the monkey mind." It is the monkey mind that keeps us awake at night, going over and over that argument with the boss. It is the monkey mind that drives us with worry and fear, making us irritable and short-tempered. The Buddhists, who have been meditating for centuries, discovered that they can drive the monkey mind out and quiet worrisome thought by repeating, rhythmically, a word or phrase, as you just practiced.

Now that you know how it feels when your sympathetic and parasympathetic nervous systems engage, you can start applying techniques in everyday life to handle the many small frustrations that become disproportionately large in the course of your normal day.

4:

How to Relax

YOU CANNOT CONTROL external events that interfere with the progress of your day—a traffic jam, a missed elevator, a lengthy on-hold time trying to reach a company by telephone. But you can control your reaction to those events quickly and easily by simply slowing down your breathing and breathing more deeply.

Next time you experience one of those minor frustrations of life that seem disproportionately annoying—a very long red light, for example—notice and pay attention to your unconscious reaction.

> You can control your reaction to stessful events by breathing slowly and deeply.

You will feel your muscles becoming tense, your breathing becoming shallow, your body having fight-or-flight symptoms such as breaking out in a sweat. All for a red light? Your conscious mind knows this makes no sense, but your unconscious mind does not—and it controls your body's reactions. So as soon as you observe those reactions—the sooner the better—slow down your breathing and breathe more deeply.

Remember, you cannot be tense and relaxed at the same time—they are incompatible feelings—so as you engage the relaxation associated with the breathing experiments, you will find your tension evaporating. It only takes a minute or two.

Repetition

ANOTHER RELAXATION TOOL is *repetition*. It can
be repetition of a sound, word, phrase, prayer or even
movement. Give this a try. Choose a word or phrase
you find soothing. Two-syllable words or phrases work
best. "Qui-et" or "re-lax" or "be-e calm" are examples.

Using a Meditative Word or Phrase

Find a comfortable place to sit. Loosen your belt
or any clothing that may be tight, constricting, or
uncomfortable. As before, rate your tension level
on a scale of 1 to 10, with 1 being very relaxed and
10 being extremely tense. Notice how you feel now.

Now silently and *slowly* say the word or phrase you
selected in a sing-song manner, stretching it out—
for example, "reeeeee-laaaaax." Repeat it over and
over in a soothing, rhythmic way. Focus your attention on the word or phrase.
When your mind wanders,
just let the distracting
thought go and bring your
attention back to the word

> *Slowly repeating a word or phrase has a lulling effect.*

or phrase. Continue to say the word or phrase
silently, slowly and rhythmically for a minute or so,
then rate your level of tension again on the scale
of 1 to 10, with 1 being very relaxed and 10 being
extremely tense.

How do you feel now? If you are like most of us, you
will have experienced an increased feeling of calm, of
distancing yourself from the usual pressures and cares
of life. As when you breathed slowly and deeply, the

repetition of the word or phrase, very slowly and again and again and again and again, has a lulling effect that removes you from the flow of ordinary stressors, focuses you inward and engages the parasympathetic nervous system.

Thinking Worries

OUR THINKING and what we tell ourselves is a strong stressor—worries. These thoughts go on constantly in our minds. Meditation gurus often say to empty your mind or make your mind blank. This is practically impossible for most people. The purpose of the meditative word or phrase is to fill the mind with these words, blocking stress-producing worries.

Our minds are both very complex and very simple. On the simple side, we can only hold one thought in the mind at a time. The purpose of the meditative word or phrase is to "fill the mind" with that single repetitive thought—to keep out the overactive monkey mind. Doing this takes a lot of practice. Drifting away from the meditative word or phrase to daily worries is inevitable. This happens to everyone, even those Buddhists sitting there thinking "OM" and saying "oooooooo-mmmmmmmm." Trying to *force* intrusive thoughts "out of your mind" only causes you to get tense, interrupting the peaceful flow that your repetitious word is producing—interfering with your calmness. So do not chastise yourself for having the thoughts. Instead, simply return your attention to the repetition of your word or phrase. It may be helpful to acknowledge the thought and then dismiss it: "Yes, I do have bills to pay, but now I am quiiii-eeet....quiiii-eeet....qui-et....qui-et."

> Worries are severe stressors for many people.

Sensing Tension

WITH PRACTICE, we can learn to relax our bodies. Actually, to be more accurate, we can learn to relax our muscles at will, which relaxes us. The first step is learning to sense tension. Many of us are chronically tense and not even aware of it. We adapt so that tension feels normal, which means you can be extremely tense and think you are relaxed. Impossible, you say? You know when you are tense? Well, try this.

Tension Exercise

Right now, make a white-knuckle fist with your left hand. Really clench it as tightly as you can and hold it. Notice how and where you feel the tension. Really study it in a dispassionate manner, as if you were a scientist analyzing the sensations.

Now, while continuing to hold your left hand in a tight fist, make a very tight fist with your *right* hand. Focus on the sensations in your now-fisted right hand and compare how your right hand feels with the way your left hand feels right now.

You probably notice that the strength of the sensations in your left hand is less than that in your right hand. You kept your left hand tightly tensed—but the sensations of tension declined quickly as a result of adaptation: you quickly adapted to the left-hand tension, and as you did, the sensations diminished. We do this all the time: sensations of tension are minimized until we hardly notice them. It is a little like walking

> Most of us are not aware of how stressed we are.

into a dark room where at first we can hardly see, but in a minute or so we can easily see because the photocells in our eyes adapted to the light—which, objectively measured, has remained the same.

When we are stressed, we quickly adapt to the sensations of tension so that we do not realize how tense we really are! This means that you may not even realize that your sympathetic nervous system is revving at full speed—but you are producing stress hormones that, when they constantly flood your body, can depress your immune system and make you feel agitated.

> Learning to sense tension is the first step to controlling it.

Sensing and Tensing

YOU CAN LEARN TO ENGAGE the relaxation response at will to quell stress—but you must be aware of the stress. The first step is to learn to sense tension. The better you become at identifying tension, the more adept you will be at purposefully relaxing that tension. Try another experiment with your fist.

Make a fist with your left hand as *lightly* as you can. Close your hand into a fist only tightly enough so you just notice the tension. Hold this lightly fisted hand for about 15 seconds or so, while objectively studying where in your hand, fingers, palm, wrist you feel the tension and just how it feels.

Next, *quickly* release the tension in your hand by opening it fast—to create a contrast in the sensations between that of tension and that of release. Compare how the hand feels when relaxed with the way it felt when tense.

The objective here is to learn to identify small degrees of tension—so you can purposefully relax your muscles *before* the tension becomes overwhelming, becoming harder to control and a greater impediment to your comfort. It is important to learn to recognize small degrees of tension, so that you can relax before stress takes over.

Systematically Tense and Relax

IT IS EASY TO LEARN to sense tension in your muscles. Working with one set of muscles at a time, such as the muscles in your face, you tense one muscle and then study the sensation of that muscle being tense—then quickly release the tension in the muscle and study the sensation of release. The self-training takes about 15 to 20 minutes, during which you progressively tense and then relax your muscles, systematically, one at a time.

After you do this self-training several times, you will become much more sensitive to sensations in your muscles and will notice tension coming on before it gets extreme. When you notice tension, you can then use a variety of techniques, which we'll cover later in this chapter, to release that tension

Progressive Relaxation

Find a place where you can be comfortable and will not be disturbed—lie down in bed, on a couch or futon, or sit in a comfortable, over-stuffed chair. Take off your shoes and loosen your belt and any tight or constricting cloth-ing. Then tense and release each muscle in the muscle groups listed below—one at a time.

With your eyes closed, tighten the muscle just enough to notice the tension. Do not tense tightly—it is important to learn to identify *slight* tension so you can intercept the stress response before it becomes full-blown. Hold the tension for about seven seconds, studying how and where you feel the tension.

Then tell yourself "relax" or "relax now" and *quickly release* the tension from each muscle, relaxing it as much as you can—and study the sensation of relaxation for ten seconds or so, comparing it with the sensation of slight tension. Then repeat the whole process a second time—light tension, quick release to relaxation, and studying the difference in how you feel. Remember, always think the "relaxation command" *just before* you quickly release the tension from the muscle.

To relax most effectively, you need to be able to identify slight tension in muscle groups throughout your body— since stress can affect you anywhere. Therefore, it is important to practice tensing and releasing all your body's muscle groups, so you can quickly determine which one is responding to stress and direct your relax command to that specific area.

Muscle Groups

Arms and hands

Hand and forearm: Make a fist.

Biceps: Bend your arm at the elbow and make a muscle.

Face and throat

Face: Squint your eyes, wrinkle your nose, and try to pull your whole face into a point at the center.

Forehead: Knit or raise your eyebrows.

Cheeks: Clench your teeth and pull the corners of your mouth toward your ears.

Nose and upper lip: With your mouth slightly open, slowly bring your upper lip down to your lower lip.

Mouth: Press the right corner of your mouth into your teeth and push the corner slowly toward the center of your mouth. Repeat with the left corner.

Lips and tongue: With your teeth slightly apart, press your lips together and push your tongue into the top of your mouth.

Chin: With your arms crossed over your chest, stick out your chin and turn it slowly as far as it will go to the left. Repeat, turning it to the right.

Neck: Push your chin into your chest, at the same time pushing your head backward into the bed or the back of your chair to create a counter-force.

Upper body

Shoulders: Attempt to touch your ears with your shoulders.

Upper back: Push your shoulder blades together and stick out your chest.

Chest: Take a deep breath.

Stomach: Pull your stomach into your spine, or push it out.

Lower body

Buttocks: Tighten your buttocks and push them into the bed or chair.

Thighs: Straighten your legs, one at a time, and tighten your thigh muscles.

Calves: Point your toes toward your head.

Toes: Curl your toes.

Again, the objective of this exercise is to learn to discriminate between the feelings of tension and relaxation so you can recognize each and transform tension into relaxation before the tension becomes severe. To be sure you are recognizing very slight tension, be careful to tense only the muscles in the area that you are studying while keeping your other muscles relaxed. For example, when tensing your biceps, you bend your arms at the elbow and make a muscle. While doing this, let your hands hang limp—because if you make a fist at the same time that you tense your biceps, you are tensing two muscle groups rather than one, and this makes it harder to study the sensation of slight tension in the biceps.

A side benefit of this self-training is that by the end of the session of tensing and relaxing your muscles systematically throughout your body, you will be very relaxed. Many people use progressive relaxation to help go to sleep at night. You might try it.

Relax Command

WHEN LEARNING SOMETHING NEW we often use self-instruction or talk ourselves through the steps, especially if they are complex, until we have it down. The relax command is a self-instruction, telling ourselves to relax. When you think the relax command and then quickly release the tension, you are doing a kind of self-programming. Release of tension is pleasurable, that is, "rewarding." By thinking "relax" and then immediately experiencing

> *When you think the relax command and then quickly release the tension, you are doing a kind of self-programming.*

the pleasure of tension release, we are "rewarding" that release and associating it with the relax command. That is how programming or conditioning works.

After you have programmed yourself with the self-training, you will be able to notice low levels of tension in various muscles, focus your attention on that tension, and think the relax command to release the tension. You could think of the human body as a kind of robot: just as you can program a robot, you can program yourself in ways like this.

Rhythmic Movement & Sounds

RHYTHMIC MOVEMENTS and repetitive sounds, such as drumming, elicit the relaxation response. As you do the same thing, over and over and over, your mind and body tune into the monotony of what you are doing and begin to focus more on the repetitiveness than on other things. Tapping your fingers repeatedly and focusing on the tapping, for example, prevents you from paying attention to what is going on around you—since the mind holds only one thought in focus at a time.

In fact, repetitive sounds are exactly what you use to elicit the relaxation response, and repetitive movements are simply another method of engaging your mind, and therefore your body, in something other than the stressors that call up the sympathetic nervous system. *Try this:*

Rock Yourself

Close your eyes, wrap your arms around yourself, and rock yourself back and forth for a minute or so. While rocking, notice how you feel.

Did you notice how lulling rocking yourself is? We all know this. We rock babies to sleep. Rocking elicits relaxation. Other repetitive movements are also lulling—for example, standing and moving your weight from one foot to the other in an even rhythm.

Repetitive sounds similarly elicit the relaxation response: chanting, drumming, a repetitive background beat such as the one used in some forms of music (see below). All of these tend to pull us into a kind of trance state. The sound of running water is also very relaxing.

Practice is important. All the methods of engaging your parasympathetic nervous system become easier as you do them more frequently. It is a good idea to practice one technique as often as you can—or several, as you discover which ones work for you under what circumstances. You will do any of the techniques more skillfully with practice, and that means you will be able to separate yourself from the destabilizing events of

Practice is important.

the day more easily, restoring your body to the balance toward which it naturally wants to gravitate.

The reason this works is that, by engaging the parasympathetic nervous system, you are encouraging the body to produce several of the healing hormones that help counteract the effects of cortisone, epinephrine and norepinephrine—the hormones of the danger-responsive fight-or-flight reflex engendered by the sympathetic nervous system.

So why not practice the relaxation response whenever you have a stress response to things in life that upset your body's homeostasis? The answer is that in many cases it is simply not practical. The reason has to do with the ongoing perceived threats of modern life—the things that provoke an all-too-constant stress response in the first place.

But you can make some headway against everyday stressors if you start small. Remember that you can elicit the relaxation response anyplace and anytime with deep breathing. Start with that. Then you might add practicing tensing and relaxing muscles one by one as you lie in bed to go to sleep. Here are some other forms of relaxation you may want to try.

Warm Baths

TAKING A WARM BATH puts us in touch with the two-thirds of our bodies made of water—the sensation of almost floating, of being surrounded by liquid and

> Warm water soothes so you don't have to "try" to relax.

supported by it, is so different from the everyday effects of fighting gravity so we can stand up and move around that a bath promotes relaxation in very short order. The warmth of the water, the warmth it brings to the room, the effect of the steam rising from the bath into the air—all of these promote a feeling of calm and of being in an environment very different from the everyday, stress-filled one.

You may enhance the effect with essential oils in the bath water, sweet-smelling candles burning in the room—many people like vanilla and lavender—or other methods of engaging your senses.

Music

LISTENING TO MUSIC is a powerful mood changer—a fact that we all know but to which we do not always pay attention. Bright, bouncy, upbeat music can pull us out of a "down" spell. In the same way, when we feel stress, calming music—whether New Age sounds, contemporary minimalist compositions, or the beautifully rhythmic and perfectly balanced works of Bach,

> We can change our moods quickly with music.

Vivaldi or Mozart—can provide us with a sense of order within the chaos of everyday life. Researchers have found that music whose tempo approximates that of our own resting heart rate can actually slow our heart to that speed and produce more-relaxed patterns of brain waves.

Try this:

Choose any music that you consider relaxing—it does not matter what type or what specific piece. Make it a selection that you already know well and like to listen to when you feel stressed. This time, instead of just letting yourself get swept away into the rhythm and tunes, focus on how you feel as the piece goes on—just as you focused on the feeling of very slight tension when you clenched your fist lightly.

Pay close attention to how you feel, what you experience, at different times during the music—you will observe just how it relaxes you, and will gain insight that may help you choose other music that you will find equally effective at combating stress.

Running Water

THE SOUND OF GENTLY FLOWING WATER can be an excellent relaxation aid. Garden fountains when you are outdoors, and tabletop fountains when you are indoors, can be tremendously calming. The gentle motion of water calls to us at a subliminal and very deep level—our bodies are about two-thirds water, and we have a visceral reaction to it.

> *Simply sit outdoors by a fountain and listen to the sound of the water moving.*

Simply sit outdoors by a fountain and listen to the sound of the water moving, the splashes it makes, the slight changes in sound as the water flows and rises and falls. Or use a tabletop fountain inside your home—you can leave it running all the time, providing a subliminally relaxing background for your everyday tasks, or you can turn it on specifically as a focus point when you are feeling stressed or having a difficult time calming down.

Some people also find white-noise generators calming—but they are not as effective for many of us as water, since the noise generation, which more or less imitates the sound of water, is at best an approximation, and some people find the sound irritating. But if you do not have a convenient location for a fountain, why not try a white-noise generator? They are small and can easily fit on, say, a bedside table, and you need not worry about spilling water if you get up during the night. The fact is that any repetitious, rhythmic sound to which you can tune in can help elicit the relaxation response by giving you something on which to focus other than the incessant demands of the "monkey mind."

Centering

THE RELAXATION RESPONSE is an excellent first line of defense against the overflow of hormones from the sympathetic nervous system when you're stressed out. It is not necessary to try to boost any specific healing hormone if you can put yourself into a wholly relaxed state in which the parasympathetic nervous system has free rein to produce its calming effects throughout your body, allowing you to separate yourself from events that you find stressful, producing a calm mental and physical state, and returning you to a "centered" feeling of homeostasis from which you will be better equipped to return to everyday activities—even if they are ones that make you feel stressed.

In addition to these ways of countering the effects of the stress hormones cortisol, adrenaline/epinephrine and norepinephrine, there are other methods of directly encouraging your body to produce larger amounts of the five healing hormones: nitric oxide, dopamine, endorphins, serotonin and oxytocin. In fact, because each healing hormone plays a different role in the body, you may want to produce more of a specific one, or several specific ones, in order to improve specific aspects of your health.

We will now look at each healing hormone in turn: what it is, what it does, how it is produced, what functions it performs, and what you can do to encourage your body to create more of it, improving specific aspects of your health and well-being.

5:

Nitric Oxide

N EVERYDAY DISCOURSE, N-O spells NO—sometimes loudly, in capital letters. But your body says Y-E-S to N-O, which is important for everyday functions as well as being the key to the helpful cardiac effects of nitroglycerin and amyl nitrate, and the sexual effects of Viagra®.

N-O is *nitric oxide*, one of several molecules formed through the combination of nitrogen and oxygen—and one that has gotten considerable bad press. Nitric oxide is a *free radical*, which means it is highly reactive with important components of the body's cells. Free radicals that proliferate can harm our bodies, and they are the reason there has been such an upsurge in interest in *antioxidants*, which are compounds that interact safely with free radicals and neutralize them. When you listen to all the arguments for taking antioxidant supplements or obtaining more antioxidants from your diet, understand that they all come down to one thing: stop the damage that free radicals can do before you suffer significant bodily harm. So nitric oxide is bad stuff, right?

Positively NO

NO, IT ISN'T. Although nitric oxide, as a free radical in the body, is implicated in cell damage, it is a powerful *vasodilator*, which widens blood vessels very effectively by causing the smooth muscle cells within vessel walls to relax. This results in significantly improved blood flow, which is precisely the mechanism on which the medicines nitroglycerin, amyl nitrate and Viagra® all rely. And this is the mechanism that makes nitric oxide a healing hormone.

Here is the science. Nitric oxide is a signaling molecule in the body—one of the few gaseous ones known. It is equivalent to, or perhaps the primary component of, the *endothelium-derived relaxing factor* or EDRF, whose discovery brought the 1998 Nobel Prize in Physiology or Medicine to researchers Robert F. Furchgott, Louis J. Ignarro and Ferid Murad. The endothelium is the thin layer of cells lining the inner surface of blood vessels—the layer affected by nitric oxide's ability to cause smooth muscle cells to relax.

> N*itric oxide has remarkable properties, of which your body takes full advantage.*

Multiple Positives

NITRIC OXIDE has remarkable properties, of which your body takes full advantage. For example, if you live at or spend time at high altitudes, you naturally produce more nitric oxide, because it helps prevent *hypoxia* or oxygen starvation—there being less oxygen in the air at higher elevations than at lower ones. It is your body's conversion of nitroglycerin and amyl nitrate to nitric oxide that produces those medicines' positive effects on your heart. Nitric oxide is good for your head, too: *minoxidil*, which slows or stops hair loss and promotes hair growth, works because it is a vasodilator that owes its effectiveness to nitric oxide. As for Viagra®, the mechanism by which it stimulates erections is directly related to the way the body uses nitric oxide.

And nitric oxide can literally be a lifesaver, as when it is used in critical-care facilities to treat newborn babies suffering from *pulmonary hypertension*—increased blood pressure that can lead to heart failure.

In fact, there are so many valuable effects of nitric oxide—despite the frequently negative attention it has received over the years in media reports—that Nobel Prize winner Ignarro founded the Nitric Oxide Society in 1996 to promote nitric-oxide research, educate people about nitric oxide, and get the word out to the public about the positive and important aspects of this biological molecule. Ignarro is something of a crusader for nitric oxide, not in respect to increasing its use but in terms of helping people understand it better. He has described it as "the body's natural way of preventing strokes and heart attacks."

> Nitric oxide is "the body's natural way of preventing strokes and heart attacks."
>
> —LOUIS J. IGNARRO, PH.D.

Supplements

AND THIS GETS TO THE HEART, so to speak, of nitric oxide as a healing hormone. Your body uses the amino acids *arginine* and, to a lesser extent, *citrulline* to produce nitric oxide. The molecule itself has a short half-life in the blood—only a few seconds—which means it is a very active substance. Its ability to boost blood flow has turned the supplement *L-arginine*—which the body converts to nitric oxide—into a popular item among bodybuilders, who want to increase the blood in their muscles during workouts in order to improve the size and shape of their bodies' blood vessels.

Supervised nitric oxide supplementation boosts strength. A University of Baylor study of people in a resistance-training program found that athletes' ability to bench-press was improved by nitric oxide. And there may be value to supplementation simply to keep people healthy as they age, because over time, the body loses its ability to produce arginine and citrulline, which means it synthesizes less nitric oxide, which in turn means the heart-helping properties of this substance are less available—which is one reason cardiovascular disease becomes more common with age.

> *Nitric oxide helps maintain normal heart function and proper blood pressure, helps fight infection, and aids your body's ability to sense pain.*

And this is not all that nitric oxide does. By signaling veins and arteries to relax and open, it improves blood circulation and lymph flow; in this way, it helps maintain normal heart function and proper blood pressure. It also helps fight infection, regulate mental and digestive functions, and aid your body's ability to sense pain, temperature and pressure. In fact, nitric oxide has so many remarkable properties that *Science* magazine named it "Molecule of the Year" in 1992.

Other NO Effects

- Helps memory by transmitting information between nerve cells in the brain
- Assists the immune system at fighting off bacteria and defending against tumors
- Reduces inflammation
- Improves sleep quality
- Boosts endurance and strength
- Assists in gastric motility

You cannot simply take a nitric oxide supplement as a pill, though, because the molecule is a gas. So researchers generally study the use of arginine—specifically *L-arginine,* one of the 20 most-common natural amino acids—to induce the body to produce more nitric oxide. This can be especially important in treating diabetes, which over time causes a reduction in blood flow to the heart, kidneys, eyes, skin and other organs. The slowing blood flow reduces oxygen levels—and oxygen is necessary to activate *nitric oxide synthase,* the enzyme that produces nitric oxide from arginine. Less oxygen means still less production of nitric oxide, which means even poorer blood flow and even higher blood pressure—which reduces oxygen still more, in a vicious cycle that is one of the significant dangers faced by diabetics. If you have diabetes, understanding this cycle can help you cope with and control your condition more effectively.

> *Researchers generally use* L-ARGININE *to induce the body to produce more nitric oxide.*

Whether you have diabetes or not, it is natural to want to know whether this healing hormone can improve your health—and, if so, how you can get more of it. Studies have shown that L-arginine supplementation has little effect on people who already have normal blood pressure—but can significantly reduce blood-pressure levels in those with borderline to high blood pressure. In other words, people with nitric oxide deficiencies are most likely to benefit from supplementation—which makes intuitive sense.

There is more to the research than that, though. In one intriguing study of 41 people with peripheral artery disease or PAD, researchers gave some of them arginine in bar form and some of them placebo bars. After two weeks, those eating two of the arginine-containing bars daily had a 66% increase in pain-free walking distance and 23% improvement in total walking distance, compared with those who ate two placebo bars or one arginine bar and one placebo bar. Another study, this one of heart-transplant patients, found that those given L-arginine supplements after surgery had increased exercise capacity.

Not So Simple

BUT AS WITH ALL HEALING HORMONES, things are not so simple. Supplementation often helps people with diminished levels of these naturally occurring substances, but *how* it helps is not always clear. One study found that L-arginine increased blood volume in the biceps—but did not improve strength. Another, done on elite college athletes, found no effect at all—which could mean that those with high cardiovascular health do not benefit from arginine supplements, while those with diminished capacity do or at least may benefit.

The sexual effects of supplementation are also uncertain: there is no doubt that Viagra® works, but although high-dose supplements of L-arginine—typically 3,000 mg daily—do seem to improve sexual response in men with erectile dysfunction, lower doses do not appear to affect blood flow to the penis. L-arginine may affect women's sexuality as well. A study published in *Journal of Sex & Marital Therapy* found that more than 70% of women who took an L-arginine supplement reported more sexual desire, more-frequent sex and orgasm, decreased vaginal dryness and greater overall sexual satisfaction.

However, supplementation may be unwise or even dangerous in people with low blood pressure, herpes, cold sores, gastric ulcer, or liver or kidney disease, because additional amounts of L-arginine can affect all those conditions. For example, people who have had cold sores or genital herpes shouldn't take L-arginine supplements, because having too much L-arginine in your system can trigger the virus that causes those conditions.

And L-arginine can have side effects, ranging from increased allergic asthmatic reactions to blood-pressure decrease. Also, those taking L-arginine may not heal as well after surgery because of changes in their blood flow.

Benefits of Arginine Supplementation

- It can help raise levels of nitric oxide and improve blood pressure and cardiac health in people with diabetes and others with borderline high blood pressure or actual hypertension.

- It helps improve exercise endurance in heart-transplant patients; and yes, high doses improve sexual response in men with erectile dysfunction.

What the research reveals is that the nitric oxide produced by arginine supplementation is a healing hormone for people deficient in this substance—but added amounts of nitric oxide, or of its precursors, probably have no significant impact.

> Physical activity is the most important way the body makes nitric oxide.
>
> — LOUIS J. IGNARRO, PH.D.

Test for Deficiency

IF YOU WANT TO FIND OUT whether you are deficient
in nitric oxide, the easiest way is with a simple saliva
test: you can buy an over-the-counter test kit at phar-
macies or online and find out for yourself. If you already
have high blood pressure or diabetes, you can assume
that you do have a nitric oxide deficiency; otherwise,
the test is an easy way to check.

And what if you do find that your body is low in
nitric oxide? Watch what you eat! As it happens, one of
the two amino acids needed to produce nitric oxide—citrulline—is difficult to get from food. The only common
food that has it in significant amounts is watermelon.

But citrulline is considerably less important for nitric oxide formation than arginine, and the good news
is that arginine is found in a wide variety of foods. See
the table on the next page for what you can do.

Other good sources of arginine to encourage your
body to make more nitric oxide include garlic, onion,
cold-water fish, eggs, chicken and green tea. Find what
you enjoy eating and eat more of it! Or try some varia-
tions in your diet—adding arginine-rich foods to what
you already eat—and your body will make more heart-
healthful nitric oxide for you.

Be careful of one thing, though: notice that the
amounts of arginine are given based on 200-calorie
servings. You can eat a lot of spinach to get to 200 calories, but only a few walnuts or cashews. So watch your
portions—you don't want to overdo the calories while
increasing your intake of arginine!

Top Arginine Boosters

(per 200-calorie serving)

- **Fresh vegetables:**
- Frozen spinach, unprepared: 3,317 milligrams
- Spirulina, raw: 3,285 mg
- Frozen spinach, cooked, boiled and drained: 2,877 mg
- Spirulina, dried: 2,861 mg
- Watercress, raw: 2,727 mg
- Pumpkin leaves, raw: 2,284
- Mustard greens, cooked, boiled and drained : 2,200 mg
- Mung beans: 1,683 mg
- **Almonds:** 812 mg
- **Dry roasted pistachios:** 738 mg
- **Flaxseed:** 721 mg
- **Roasted sunflower seeds:** 715 mg
- **Walnuts:** 697 mg
- **Cashews:** 607 mg
- **Pecans:** 341 mg

Exercise Is Important

FOOD IS NOT THE ONLY WAY to get your body to make more nitric oxide. In fact, it is not even the most important way, according to Dr. Ignarro. What matters more? Exercise! Dr. Ignarro puts it simply: "Physical activity is the most important way the body makes nitric oxide." The heart beats faster when you exercise; this boosts blood flow through the arteries; and that stimulates production of nitric oxide.

It is true that if you have very low levels of nitric oxide, you may need actual supplements of L-arginine, but be sure to discuss this with your doctor before starting the supplement. A daily dose of up to nine grams of L-arginine—taken three grams at a time, three times per day—is generally considered safe, but not for everyone and not under all circumstances. And supplementation is really needed only if your body has very low levels of this important healing hormone.

You may wonder why there is nothing in scientific literature about nitric oxide's use as laughing gas. The answer is that while laughing gas is a mixture of nitrogen and oxygen, it is a different combination. It is not nitric oxide but *nitrous* oxide—shown chemically as N_2O. Nitrous oxide has been used as an anesthetic since it was first employed by a dentist in 1844.

Some effects attributed to nitrous and nitric oxide are indeed similar, such as a boost in sexual pleasure—but the mechanisms are very different. The phrase "laughing gas" applies strictly to *nitrous* oxide.

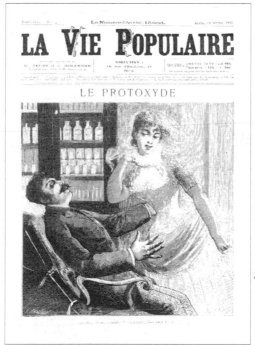

A 19th-century French impression of nitrous oxide's sexual effects.

6:

Dopamine

WOULDN'T IT BE WONDERFUL if there were other healing hormones, besides nitric oxide, that you could encourage your body to produce simply by doing certain things or eating certain foods—no medicines or supplements required? Good news: dopamine—sometimes labeled a "feel-good" chemical because it is what makes us experience pleasure when we engage in rewarding behavior—is another healing hormone that your body produces in greater quantities based on what you eat.

What makes dopamine a healing hormone? Like nitric oxide, it is a neurotransmitter, which is a chemical released by nerve cells to send messages to other nerve cells. Dopamine must be important, since it is produced in several areas of the brain, not just in one place; and there are five different known types of dopamine receptors, labeled from D_1 to D_5.

Reward-Driven Learning

SCIENTIFIC and medical details aside, dopamine is tremendously important in the brain system for *reward-driven learning*. When we engage in rewarding or pleasurable behavior, our bodies increase dopamine production and we "feel good." Every single type of reward that researchers have studied raises the level of dopamine transmission in the brain. Dopamine affects movement: a certain amount is necessary for normal motion of our limbs and body, and disturbances in dopamine production or use cause motion to be jerky or irregular. Dopamine affects emotions: the higher the level of dopamine, or the more responsive the brain is to dopamine, the more likely a person is to be sensitive to incentives and rewards. Dopamine affects memory: it helps protect against noises and distractions, making memory-intensive planning and problem solving easier.

And dopamine is involved in the experience of pleasure—any kind of pleasure. Dopamine release produces a cascade of feelings that we identify as pleasurable whenever we are exposed to an event, substance or situation that makes us feel god. This is one of our body's many

> **D**opamine affects movement, emotions, memory and the experience of pleasure—any kind of pleasure.

elegant feedback loops: pleasure leads to more dopamine production, and more dopamine leads to greater feelings of pleasure, which leads us to want even more of the pleasure that induced the dopamine increase in the first place, and so on. This is why dopamine can be thought of as a body-produced feel-good drug.

When our bodies do not produce enough dopamine, we feel, in a word, rotten. Symptoms may include depression, inability to focus, loss of motor control, diminished sex drive, cravings for or addictions to pleasure-giving substances, lack of motivation, compulsion, and a generalized loss of satisfaction with life. Dopamine is powerful stuff.

Unfortunately for all of us living with the everyday pressures of modern life, many of the things we face day in and day out deplete dopamine levels—explaining why so many people have a general feeling of "dragginess" or anomie so much of the time. Among dopamine depleters are stress, lack of sleep, poor diet, saturated-fat intake, and alcohol. Medication use can also reduce dopamine levels—certain antidepressants, in particular, are known to cause a reduction in dopamine, and this can produce a vicious cycle: someone who feels depressed takes an antidepressant that depletes dopamine, so the person feels even more depressed and wants more of the antidepressant.

Serious Conditions

DOPAMINE is so important to our emotional balance and normal function that modest changes in the body's production of it can have serious consequences. Schizophrenia, for example, is partly caused by a dopamine imbalance—elevated levels in a part of the brain called the *mesolimbic pathway* and reduced levels in a different part, the *prefrontal cortex*. Among other conditions related to reduced dopamine activity are attention deficit-hyperactivity disorder, known as ADHD, and restless legs syndrome.

And then there is Parkinson's disease, which causes tremors and impaired motion. Parkinson's is age-related and is directly caused by a drop in dopamine, specifically by the loss of neurons that secrete dopamine in a part of the brain called the *substantia nigra*. Anytime dopamine production is disturbed, the effects can be serious.

And "disturbed" does not necessarily mean "reduced." Lower dopamine is more common than too-high dopamine, but if you *do* have too much dopamine, you can experience high anxiety levels, panic attacks, hyperactivity and paranoia. Dopamine is also responsible for the attractiveness of drugs such as cocaine and methamphetamine, which stimulate dopamine production and thus engage the self-reinforcing loop of higher dopamine production leading to increased desire for the substance that has caused dopamine levels to rise.

For most of us, though, it is reduced dopamine levels that produce a feeling of malaise and generalized discomfort, a sense that all is not right with the world, a feeling of uneasiness and of trouble coping with life—even a reluctance to get out of bed in the morning. The notion of a dopamine supplement

> D*opamine is responsible for the attractiveness of drugs such as cocaine and methamphetamine.*

is therefore attractive: just add dopamine to life and everything will get better.

Unfortunately, this does not work. Dopamine *can* be given as a supplement—although only intravenously— but when administered that way, it does not affect the central nervous system and does not improve mood. It does, however, save lives. Dopamine increases heart rate and blood pressure, and is therefore used in patients with serious heart failure and, sometimes, those with kidney failure or the life-threatening blood infection *septicemia*. But these are extreme uses that usually occur in intensive-care units of hospitals, where the patient can be closely monitored and the dopamine dose carefully adjusted as necessary.

Blood-Brain Barrier

TO RAISE THE LEVELS of dopamine in the brain, what is needed is a way to cross the *blood-brain barrier*, a physiological process that significantly restricts the passage of most substances from the bloodstream into the brain. Dopamine cannot cross this barrier, which is why dopamine supplementation does not affect mood or feelings despite the power of this healing hormone to save lives. However, a *precursor* of dopamine, known as *L-Dopa* or *levodopa*, does cross this barrier, and it is this chemical that is now the standard treatment for Parkinson's disease and certain other dopamine-related conditions. The clinical use of L-Dopa on this basis was devised by a medical scientist named George C. Cotzias. His first study of the effective use of L-Dopa for patients with Parkinson's was published in 1968; it was in 1970 that the Food and Drug Administration approved the use of L-Dopa for this purpose

But even the use of L-Dopa to raise dopamine levels is not simple. Cotzias was not the first to try it. Dopamine was proven to be a neurotransmitter in the brain in the 1950s by Swedish scientist Arvid Carlsson, whose work with dopamine made him one of three recipients of the Nobel Prize in Physiology or Medicine in 2000. A number of doctors treated Parkinson's patients with L-Dopa after Carlsson's discovery and his subsequent work showing the relationship between dopamine levels in the brain and movement control.

But injections of L-Dopa in amounts sufficient to relieve Parkinson's symptoms had such high levels of toxicity that they were considered impractical as a treatment. What Cotzias did was to develop a protocol that started with very small L-Dopa doses, given orally rather than by injection, and administered every two hours under very close observation. He

> The use of L-Dopa to raise dopamine levels is not simple.

gradually increased the dose of L-Dopa and was eventually able to raise it to a clinically effective level.

The Standard Method

THIS HUGE BREAKTHROUGH for Parkinson's treatment, which remains the standard method of caring for
patients with the disease, shows that there is nothing
simple or straightforward about trying to raise dopamine
levels through supplementation. But dopamine is so
important for health and so closely tied to feelings of
pleasure and relaxation, to a sense that life is good and
all is right with the world—or at least not bad—that
the temptation to raise dopamine with supplements is
understandably strong. And there is a nonprescription
way to do this, using a herbal preparation called *mucuna
pruriens* or *velvet bean*. This is generally taken as an
800-milligram dose that may contain up to 120 milligrams of L-Dopa.

But although this is a legal supplement available
without prescription—unlike more-potent doses of
L-Dopa, which are prescription-only—it is definitely
not for everyone, and not to be taken without talking to your doctor first. Dopamine is, after all, a strong
psychoactive substance—that is its whole "reason for
being," so to speak. Anything that raises dopamine levels affects personality and behavior; and this of course is
just what anyone considering a supplement wants. But
the side effects of consum-
ing L-Dopa, even in modest
quantities, are not to be
trifled with: nausea, hypertension, cardiac arrhythmia,
gastrointestinal bleeding,
hallucinations and even
narcolepsy have been reported. The more-serious side
effects are uncommon when L-Dopa is taken in modest
doses, but they *do* occur.

> The side effects of
> consuming L-Dopa
> are not to be trifled
> with.

There are better ways to raise dopamine levels. The key to healing hormones is that they are *naturally occurring substances*, which means that your body creates them. So instead of trying to increase them by bringing in chemicals from outside in the form of supplements, you can do things that cause your own body, naturally, to increase its production of these hormones.

Be Active

IN THE CASE OF DOPAMINE, there are some things to do and some *not* to do. In addition to eating more foods that contain the dopamine precursor *tyrosine*, an amino acid, another thing you can do to increase your body's dopamine production is to exercise. This may seem surprising if exercise is not already part of your daily routine. If you do not exercise, one likely reason may be that it makes you ache and feel bad. How can it possibly release a feel-good hormone such as dopamine?

The answer is that length and intensity of exercise make a difference—a fact well known to athletes and those who enjoy extended exercise regularly. To stimulate brain activity enough to cause the brain to produce significant amounts of neurotransmitters, you need to exercise for at least 20 to 30 minutes, and keep your heart rate elevated while working out. If this gives you pleasure, dopamine will encourage you to do more of it.

> To stimulate brain activity enough to cause the brain to produce significant amounts of neurotransmitters, you need to exercise for at least 20 to 30 minutes.

Reward for Sex

SPEAKING OF PLEASURE, one way to raise dopamine levels is with sexual activity. And the effect is more immediate than with exercise—that is, other forms of exercise. Raised dopamine levels are a way that the body rewards us humans, and other animals, for engaging in actions that perpetuate the species. But few people are likely to seek out additional sexual contact for this reason—there are plenty of other motivations for sex than a rise in the production of neurotransmitters. Nevertheless, feel free to add a dopamine boost to your reasons for wanting more sex.

Food, Too

FOOD IS AS NATURAL a part of life as sex, and as already mentioned, eating certain foods can have an effect on dopamine production: foods rich in the amino acid *tyrosine* encourage the body to produce more dopamine. Generally, fresh fruits, vegetables, whole grains and legumes all lead the body to make more dopamine. One champion food source that is easy to eat anytime is a ripe banana. But foods are also an area where there are things *not* to do. Fats and cholesterol tend to lower dopamine levels, and so do high quantities of sugar—so avoiding sugar-added foods may be good not only for your waistline but also for your brain's hormone production.

Like nitric acid, dopamine is derived from amino acids—in this case, just one, *tyrosine*. So eating more foods that provide tyrosine will result in your body making more dopamine. And there are plenty of tyrosine-rich foods, including almonds, sesame seeds, dairy products, bananas, and avocados.

Selected Tyrosine Boosters

(per 200-calorie serving)

- **Spirulina, raw:** 2,046 mg
- **Soy protein isolate:** 1,907 to 2,008 mg
- **Egg white:** 1,904 mg
- **Low-fat cottage cheese:** 1,833 mg
- **Salmon:** 1,744 mg
- **Turkey, light meat:** 1,610 to 1,771 mg
- **Shrimp:** 1,620 mg
- **Mustard greens:** 1,587 mg
- **Pork:** 1,579 mg
- **Fat-free cream cheese:** 1,528 mg
- **Orange roughy:** 1,522 mg

Sugar

HOWEVER, as anyone who loves sugar is well aware, cutting back on sugar-containing foods makes you feel worse, not better. This is where the complexity of dopamine response comes in. As with drugs such as cocaine, sugar does provide many people with immediate short-lived gratification and enhanced dopamine production, which then produces a craving for more of the substance—the drug or food—that brought the heightened pleasure. This is how the dopamine cycle can turn negative.

> *Eating fresh fruits, vegetables, whole grains and legumes leads the body to make more dopamine.*

The key here, though, is that the pleasure boost from sugar is temporary and is followed fairly quickly by a significant drop in enjoyment—the well-known "sugar high" and "sugar low." Where dopamine is concerned, sugar is not the only substance that causes this: caffeine tends to raise dopamine levels temporarily, but the effect soon wears off—one reason people who drink caffeinated coffee often drink it almost constantly.

Vitamin Boosters

EXERCISE AND EATING tyrosine-rich foods are the best methods of encouraging your body to keep making dopamine at high enough levels to counteract the effects of dopamine reducers such as lack of sleep and the stress response.

After all this, if you do want to consider supplements, there is a better approach than using L-Dopa: take vitamins that stimulate dopamine production. There are four of these. Vitamin A—found in fish, liver, dairy products and eggs—has, among its other functions, the stimulation of dopamine production. Vitamin B_6 is tied to amino-acid metabolism, which includes production of dopamine. And two vitamins that are strong antioxidants—protecting cells against oxidative stress and helping the body remove toxins— are vitamins C and E, both of which are important for hormone production and conversion. In fact, doses of vitamin E are sometimes given as a nutritional supplement to patients being treated with L-Dopa for Parkinson's disease. Vitamins C and E tend to stimulate each other's effects, so they are best taken together.

It is a common misconception that taking large doses of vitamins will somehow cause the body to do a lot more of the things with which the vitamins are associated. Most of the time, this is not true. Vitamin supplements are used by the body to the extent that there is an existing deficiency, and additional amounts are simply excreted. So there is no reason to take very large vitamin doses in the hope of stimulating a large amount of dopamine production. But vitamin supplements up to the recommended daily intake can help keep your body in balance, producing enough dopamine to enhance your mood and counteracting the effects of all those "downers" in daily life.

7:

Endorphins

WHAT DO PETTING YOUR DOG, eating chili peppers, laughing, and getting a massage have in common? They are all ways of getting your body to produce more of the healing hormones called *endorphins*. Endorphins are powerful calming chemicals that produce a deep-seated feeling of well-being. In fact, the very word "endorphin" means "endogenous morphine"—which is to say, "a morphine-like substance that originates inside the body"—although endorphins are not actually the same as morphine.

Paradoxical Healers

ENDORPHINS, like the other healing hormones, are neurotransmitters, substances that facilitate communication within the brain—in effect, the chemical messengers through which our brains tell our bodies which sensations to experience and to what degree. But there is something surprising about the feelings of well-being produced by endorphins: they go hand-in-hand with endorphins' pain-relieving ability. Endorphins are our bodies' natural pain relievers.

Where Produced

ENDORPHINS are produced by the *hypothalamus*, a portion of the brain located just above the brain stem, and by the *pituitary gland,* a pea-sized structure that is not part of the brain but that is found at the bottom of the hypothalamus at the brain's base—and is connected to the hypothalamus by a tube called the *pituitary stalk.*

Triggered by Pain

ENDORPHINS' production is triggered by stress and pain. And there are at least 20 different types of endorphins, which is why they are usually written about in the plural—unlike nitric oxide and dopamine, which are written as singular nouns. Endorphins interact with the body's *opioid receptors*—sites that provide pain relief. The receptors are widely distributed in the brain and also found in the digestive tract and spinal cord. And there are four major types of opioid receptors, which have different but sometimes overlapping functions.

This is why endorphins have a wide variety of effects and are responsible for some well-known differences among people, such as the fact that individuals who suffer the same objectively measured amount of pain may respond to it very differently.

> Endorphins are responsible for some well-known differences among people, such as the fact that individuals who suffer the same amount of pain may respond to it very differently.

We all know someone who seems unusually sensitive to pain or unusually indifferent to it. Endorphins are the reason for these differing responses: some people's bodies naturally produce more endorphins and some produce less.

The key to the positive feelings created by endorphins lies partly in their relationship to the healing hormone, dopamine. When the body releases endorphins, which bind to opioid receptors, two things happen. First, neurotransmitters that cause the feeling of pain are blocked. And second, the brain creates more do-pamine—which, as we have seen, produces feelings of pleasure.

Pain and Fun

ENDORPHINS are a paradox. Our bodies make more of them when we are in pain—because they relieve pain. But our bodies also make more of them when we are happy. Endorphin production responds to laughter or, surprisingly, even the *anticipation* of laughter—or fun.

Endorphin-Promoting Activities

Laugh—Laugh a Lot!

WATCH A FUNNY MOVIE. There are many of them, for all tastes. Find one that matches yours. It could be a classic comedy. It could be a film full of pratfalls and custard pies. It could have snappy dialogue. It could have no dialogue at all—some silent movies are hilarious. It could feature a famed comedian, such as Charles Chaplin. Or a group, like the characters in *Animal House*. It could be by a well-known director or an unknown. It could have sight gags or witty dialogue. It could be a cartoon—full-length or short. It could even be *unintentionally* funny, one of those movies that are "so bad they're good."

> Your body produces endorphins when you laugh.

Not into movies? Act silly with your friends. Pose
with statues. Snap photos in ridiculous positions.
Repeat bad jokes or make up new ones. Watch TV
together and laugh at shows *and* commercials. Eat food
in a silly way—try soup with a fork—and laugh about it.
Wear clothing backwards. Have a funny-face contest.
Watch ridiculous YouTube videos—there are thousands and thousands and thousands of them. Play board
games backwards.

A fascinating study by two California scientists, Lee
S. Berk of Loma Linda University and Stanley A. Tan
of Oakcrest Health Research Institute, looked at endorphins and laughter in a very surprising way. Berk and
Tan, working with 16 healthy male volunteers, found
that *anticipating* laughter was enough to raise endorphin
levels: they told the men in advance whether or not
they would be in a group enjoying laughter-provoking
experiences, and found that the bodies of those who
would be in that group increased endorphin production
in anticipation of the amusement to come.

This is a marvelous finding, because it means you
can raise your body's level of endorphins even before
going to a funny movie or a comedy club. You just
have to make the decision to attend and anticipate the
outing, and your body will, in effect, get ready to be
amused by producing more
endorphins—and then will
produce even more when you
have the laughter-provoking
experience. How you do this is

> *Your body gets ready to be amused by producing more endorphins.*

by expecting funny things. Think about them. Imagine
what they might be. Think of the fun you will have.
The silly things you will see. How much you will enjoy
yourself.

"Runner's High"

PEOPLE WHO WORK OUT INTENSELY, whether as runners or in other high-intensity sports, often experience this euphoric feeling, and many know that endorphins cause it. Some call it "being in the zone." Exercise—intense and sustained—is one way of getting your body to produce more endorphins. In effect, you are causing stress in your body and thus getting it to produce pain-minimizing relaxation substances. But what you are really doing—if you are one of the people who experience "runner's high"—is substituting one form of stress, a positive one, for another, negative one.

Here's why. Remember that stress is a necessary element of life: the right amount of it, not too little and not too much, is adaptive, helping us cope with changes in our external environment. People who enjoy intense exercise often speak of it as a stress reliever, and for them, it is.

The *mental* and *emotional* stress response that so many of us live with day in and day out, which leads to the production of fight-or-flight hormones such as cortisol and epinephrine, can be overcome naturally by subjecting the body to the *physical* stress of a good workout—which causes production of endorphins, which counteract the effects of fight-or-flight hormones. This is an elegant way of using a desirable, self-induced stress response to counteract the undesirable one that occurs because of external factors such as your job, traffic, financial issues, family matters and so forth.

Be Sexy

NOT EVERYONE who exercises will ever experience "runner's high," and in fact many people find exercise mentally, emotionally and physically stressful. So they will probably not exercise regularly and intensely enough to boost endorphin production sufficiently to benefit from this healing hormone. If you are one of those people and would like a different endorphin-boosting activity suggestion, try sex! Indeed, sex, which raises dopamine levels, also increases the production of endorphins—which, if you think about it, makes sense, since biologically, sex represents yet another kind of body stress.

This does not just mean engaging in actual inter-course—it means *connecting*. Give hugs. Give pats. Have public displays of affection. Caress each other—within appropriate limits—while walking on the street or eating in a restaurant. Touch each other for any rea-son or no reason at all. Put your arms around your part-ner while walking—or at home while sitting together. Eat meals next to each other, not across the table, so your bodies can touch. Enjoy the closeness!

Massage and More

OUR BODIES release endorphins when we are stressed—and also when we are relaxed. Get a massage—or give one! Massages relax us and our bodies respond with endorphin release. Acupuncture works, too—scientific studies have found it to be effective when done by a skilled practitioner who targets certain specific acu-puncture points.

There is also pseudoscience, totally unproven and with only anecdotal evidence to back it up, that may nevertheless boost your endorphin level—activities such as "tapping," a self-administration of something like acupuncture, but without needles. Instructions can be found on the Internet; and even though there are only personal testimonials and little hard scientific evidence, it seems to work for *some* people and certainly has potential if you believe in it.

> You can boost endorphins as much as you like with exercise, sex, laughter, and all the chili peppers you can consume, and the only physical effects will be positive ones.

What is interesting is how many ways we can induce our bodies to boost endorphin production: intense exercise, meditation, massage and acupuncture seem to have very little to do with each other, but in terms of the body's response to them, they can all be effective as endorphin boosters.

Pet Your Pet

JOHANNES ODENDAAL, a South African psychologist, physiologist and veterinarian, found that dog and human interaction improved the happiness hormones in both humans and pets.

After just thirty minutes of interaction, multiple hormones connected with happiness and well-being—not only endorphins but also dopamine and oxytocin—increased significantly, while stress hormones, such as cortisol, fell. This is why dogs—and sometimes cats—are used in healthcare settings. "When therapy dogs are at patient bedsides, we see a noticeable change in patients," said Bonnie Petrie, a geriatric care manager in Fort Lauderdale, Florida. "They smile, relax, and it opens up dialogue. It also makes the hospital feel less like an institution and provides a more nurturing environment." Nurture yourself with your own pet therapy—it's good for your pet, too!

Listen to Music

LISTEN TO whatever form of music you like, whenever
you want to—not as background but as a point of focus.
Just tuning into the rhythm of the music, listening to
it while excluding other sounds, transports you out of
everyday cares and into a world where melodies flow
naturally and, as a result, endorphins flow as well.

You can use music to calm yourself or invigorate
yourself—what matters is that you enjoy it and focus on
it while it is playing. Result: more endorphins!

Foods to Try

FOODS THAT cause pleasure as well as ones that cause
pain are effective endorphin boosters. This is part of
the paradox of endorphins: they are released when
enjoyable things happen and also when the body needs
calming, healing and repair. So you can use a favorite
food that gives you pleasure to increase your endorphin
production. But you can also use one whose effects the
body perceives as painful!

Dark Chocolate

EATING DARK CHOCOLATE is known to cause endorphin levels to rise, and this may explain why many
people find chocolate consumption comforting and
why so many of us crave chocolate when we are feeling stressed. A chemical found in chocolate, theobromine, is a kind of natural antidepressant: it triggers
the release of endorphins and is largely responsible for
chocolate's mood-boosting effects. Theobromine is
a natural component of the cacao bean, from which
chocolate is made. Certain chocolate bars, hot cocoa

and chocolate ice cream have particularly high levels of theobromine—a point worth remembering when giving or receiving chocolate at Valentine's Day! In fact, the whole association between Valentine's Day and chocolate reinforces the notion of a feel-good, loving-connection holiday.

Spicy Foods

SPICY FOODS TRIGGER endorphin release. The spicier the better, by the way! Spiciness is not really a taste sensation but an experience of pain. In particular, *capsaicin*, the chemical that makes chili peppers "hot," binds to pain receptors of the nerve cells in the mucous membranes of the mouth and nose. This produces nerve impulses that pass into the brain and create a painful burning sensation—to which the brain responds by releasing endorphins as a pain-soothing analgesic.

G inseng, vanilla and lavender may raise endorphin levels in some people.

If you like to eat spicy foods, you are ahead of the game where endorphin production is concerned—although you may have to eat even more of them to get the same boost that a smaller amount will bring to someone who does not customarily eat "hot" foods.

Ginseng

GINSENG IS A SHORT, slow-growing perennial plant with fleshy roots—there are eleven different species. It is harvested as a herb. The herbs consist of a light-colored, fork-shaped root, a relatively long stalk and green leaves with an oval shape. Many people believe that

ginseng restores and enhances normal well-being—with
the result that ginseng is a very popular herbal supplement. And it does seem to help balance the production of fight-or-flight hormones. Also, some runners
and other athletes believe it increases physical endurance and helps them attain a "runner's high."

Pleasing Aromas

BREATHING PLEASING AROMAS such as vanilla and
lavender is generally considered to boost your mood.
Both have been used experimentally to treat people
who are depressed, anxious or feeling highly stressed.
Burning vanilla-scented candles or using a lavender-oil
diffuser may lead your body to produce more endorphins and counteract stress. Psychologically, it may simply be that your focus on the preparation of a method of
producing vanilla or lavender scent takes your mind off
your stressors and helps you unwind—but whether the
effect is psychological, physical or both, it is worthwhile
to find out whether it works for you.

Another way to expose yourself to relaxing aromas
that may boost your endorphins is by planting flowers
with intense odors, such as gardenias, along the walk
leading into your house. This will give you a strong
dose of their odor every time you walk in or out. Or you
may enjoy the delicate
scent of lily-of-the-valley.
Other wonderful picks
include sweet alyssum,
sweet pea, and roses.

> A desirable, self-induced stress response can counteract the undesirable one that occurs because of external factors.

Each time you step out of
your house or come home you will be bathed in wonderful endorphin-promoting armomas.

Avoid Opioid Meds

WHAT DOES NOT WORK for increased endorphin production is the use of opioid medications. Remember that the word "endorphin" means "endogenous morphine," which points to a pain reliever produced by the body; and endorphins work by attaching themselves—that is, binding—to the body's opioid receptors.

These are precisely the receptors to which codeine, morphine and other pain relievers, such as Vicodin®, also bind. But those are *exogenous* substances, which means they originate outside the body—"exogenous" is the opposite of "endogenous." Exogenous opioids have an effect that endogenous ones do not, and that is addiction.

What this means is simply that both endorphins and opioids are chemicals that relieve pain and can make you feel good. But ingesting exogenous substances eventually leads to tolerance that requires ever-higher doses for the same effect—and discontinuing those substances can produce severe withdrawal symptoms. None of this happens with endogenous morphine—that is, with endorphins, which are created internally by the body. You can boost endorphins as much as you like with exercise, sex, laughter, and all the chili peppers you can consume, and the only physical effects will be positive ones.

8:

Serotonin

S EROTONIN is the neurotransmitter that makes you feel happy, comfortable and content—so relaxed, in fact, that it is important for getting a good night's sleep. Sometimes thought of as the "happy hormone," serotonin is more than that, because the happiness it conveys is not of the ha-ha type but is more a feeling of relaxation and contentment, a sense that all is right with the world. Think of serotonin as a sort of anti-stress or de-stressing hormone and you will have it about right.

Turkey, Milk and More

THIS IS A HORMONE whose production most people increase all the time, whether they intend to or not. Serotonin is made from the amino acid *tryptophan*, which is found in protein and which we humans—being protein eaters—consume in considerable quantities. If you have ever overindulged in turkey at Thanksgiving or drunk a glass of warm milk at bedtime, you have unwittingly boosted your serotonin level. Both turkey and milk are good sources of tryptophan, and the more tryptophan in your body, the more serotonin you produce. Plenty of other protein sources are filled with tryptophan, too.

Tryptophan Boosters

(per 200-calorie serving)

- **Soy protein isolate:** 685 mg
- **Egg white:** 673 mg
- **Alaska king crab:** 607 mg
- **Halibut:** 593 mg
- **Shrimp:** 588 mg
- **Lobster:** 582 mg
- **Blue crab:** 578 mg
- **Crayfish:** 577 mg
- **Pork:** 571 mg
- **Dungeness crab:** 566 mg
- **Duck:** 543 mg

Mood Modulator

SEROTONIN is a key mood modulator. When your body has an optimal amount, you feel pleasantly balanced and at peace with your environment. Unfortunately, many people have either too little serotonin or too much. Since serotonin is a kind of anti-stress hormone, it is no surprise that prolonged periods of the fight-or-flight response depress its production. Nor is perceived stress the only culprit.

Quite a few elements of everyday modern life are thought to pull down serotonin levels, although there is disagreement about the relative importance of these situations. The list of serotonin inhibitors is a long one, from deficiency of tryptophan—on which everyone agrees—to niacin and/or progesterone deficiency and/or deficiencies in other vitamins and minerals, lack of exposure to sunlight, overexposure to plastics and chemicals, insulin resistance, as well as genetic factors.

Serotonin deficiency results in a large number of symptoms that are all too common nowadays. Most of them are depressive in nature even if they do not advance to the level of full-scale clinical depression. Too-low amounts of serotonin can lead to anxiety, excessive worrying, pessimism, suicidal thoughts and tendencies, low self-esteem, and a strong negative reaction to dark weather. Free-floating fear—not directed at any specific situation—can occur when serotonin levels are too low. So can panic, phobias and obsession.

> *When your body has an optimal amount of serotonin, you feel pleasantly balanced and at peace with your environment.*

Even people who do not have such strong reactions may experience irritation, impatience, repetitive thinking, anger and aggression. Since serotonin relaxes us and helps us sleep, too-low levels can produce too-light sleep or insomnia. Low serotonin production is also associated with sugar cravings, chronic pain, and other symptoms—the list goes on and on. This healing hormone is particularly powerful.

Since it *is* a healing hormone, though, and one whose production it is particularly easy to increase through food consumption, it is tempting to "stock up" on serotonin so that you have even more of it than you absolutely need—the idea being to avoid the unpleas-

ant symptoms of serotonin deficiency and feel even better, even more relaxed and at peace, than you otherwise
would.

The Golden Mean

UNFORTUNATELY, trying to increase serotonin beyond a certain level does not work. As with so many
bodily processes, there is a Golden Mean for keeping
our bodies in balance. Overproduction of serotonin is
a problem because it will make you feel sleepy at inap-
propriate times. It may be fine to collapse into inertia
after a large Thanksgiving feast or a dinner built around
generous servings of chicken—which, like turkey, is
high in tryptophan.

However, this level of relaxation will not help you
do your best at work if, for example, you overindulge
at lunch in foods that boost serotonin production. In
fact, most of us have experienced a kind of "afternoon
sluggishness" of this sort from time to time. Serotonin
is to blame, and the consequences of *regular* diminished
afternoon productivity are certainly not pleasant ones
in the workplace.

Worse, an overproduction of serotonin can be
significantly more dangerous. A condition called *se-*
rotonin syndrome can occur when your body has too
much serotonin—and it is nothing to trifle with. At its
most severe, it can be fatal. Even in less-serious form,
serotonin syndrome produces a long list of unpleasant
symptoms.

Serotonin Syndrome

- Shivering
- Heavy sweating
- Diarrhea
- Confusion
- Agitation
- Rapid heart rate
- Increased blood pressure
- Loss of muscle coordination

Things get even worse as serotonin syndrome progresses: more-serious symptoms can include high fever, muscle rigidity, irregular heartbeat, seizures, and unconsciousness.

Don't worry: you will not get serotonin syndrome from your Thanksgiving turkey! This healing hormone is produced by the body in several areas: serotonin made in the brain and spinal cord helps regulate attention, behavior and body temperature; serotonin made in the intestines helps regulate blood flow, breathing and digestion. What throws production into overdrive is not what the body itself does but what happens when you introduce substances from outside the body—so-called *exogenous* substances. Exogenous methods of boosting serotonin production are detrimental in ways that increasing your body's own production is not.

> **S**erotonin syndrome is usually caused by combinations of medications.

Serotonin syndrome is usually caused by medications—
most of the time, by two or more
medicines taken in combination.
Some of the drugs that can lead
to serotonin syndrome are well-
known and quite widely used.
They are the antidepressants
called SSRIs or *selective serotonin reuptake inhibitors*, including citalaporam, best known
as Celexa®; fluoxetine, sold as
Prozac® and Sarafem®; fluvox-
amine, sold as Luvox®; parox-
etine, best known as Paxil®; and
sertraline, sold as Zoloft®. Other
drugs associated with serotonin
syndrome are SNRIs or *serotonin
and norepinephrine reuptake inhibitors*, including trazodone, sold as
Desyrel®, Oleptro® and under
other brand names, and venla-
faxine, best known as Effexor®.

Serotonin Syndrome

*S*erotonin syndrome
can be caused by
taking one of these
antidepressants along
with migraine-fight-
ing medications such
as carbamazepine,
sold as Tegretol®,
or valproic acid, sold
as Depakene®; pain
medicines includ-
ing cyclobenzaprine,
sold as Flexeril®, and
tramadol, sold as
Ultram®; the mood
stabilizer lithium,
sold as Lithobid®; or
anti-nausea medi-
cines such as meto-
clopramide, sold as
Reglan®, and ondan-
setron, sold as Zo-
fran®.

Other forms of antidepressants may be involved, too.
Among these are *tricyclic anti-
depressants*, such as amitriptyline, sold as Tryptomer®,
Elavil® and under other names, and nortriptyline, best
known as Pamelor®; and MAOIs or *monoamine oxidase
inhibitors*, including isocarboxazid, sold as Marplan®,
and phenelzine, sold as Nardil®.

Serotonin syndrome is unlikely to be caused by
taking just one of these medicines, but where the situation gets complicated is that it can occur in people
who take any of these antidepressants *plus* certain other
prescription medicines—or even some over-the-counter

products or herbal supplements, which patients do not always think of as medications and may not tell their doctors they are using.

Cough Medicines and Herbs

OVER-THE-COUNTER cough and cold medicines that contain a commonly used and very well-known cough suppressant called *dextromethorphan* are among the drugs whose interaction with antidepressants can lead to serotonin syndrome—that is, brands such as Delsym®, Robitussin DM® and others. And what about herbs? Taking ginseng or St. John's wort along with another serotonin-raising substance can bring on serotonin syndrome. So can use of illicit drugs such as amphetamines, cocaine, LSD, and MDMA—often known as Ecstasy.

And various herbal preparations may interact with *each other* to bring on serotonin syndrome—even if you do not take an antidepressant, it is theoretically possible to develop the syndrome by taking sufficient quantities of, say, St. John's wort plus ginseng plus an over-the-counter (OTC) cold medicine. *Any* combination of drugs known to raise serotonin levels may lead to serotonin syndrome, and too-high doses of a *single* drug may do so as well—this happens most often when people deliberately take higher-than-prescribed doses of antidepressants.

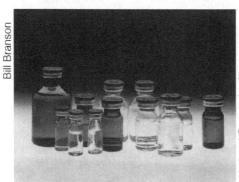

Bill Branson

National Cancer Institute

Medication bottles

Dangerous Combinations

YOU MIGHT THINK that serotonin syndrome is simple to avoid by just taking prescribed medications in the proper amounts, but things are a bit more complicated than that because of the fact that non-prescription drugs and herbal supplements may also cause the syndrome. And it is unreasonable to expect everyone who is on one of the SSRIs and who has a cold to remember not to use dextromethorphan-containing OTC medications...

> *Taking higher than prescribed doses of antidepressants can raise serotonin levels and bring on serotonin syndrome.*

or to avoid using ginger in an attempt to treat arthritis or diarrhea, as some people do.

Ideally, your doctor will know every medicine, both prescription and OTC, that you take, and all herbal supplements as well, and will be able to alert you to possible interactions such as serotonin syndrome; ideally, your pharmacist will also be sensitive to the situation. But in the real world as opposed to an ideal one, you yourself need to be aware of what you put into your body and what interactive effects may result—and take action if something is not right.

Fortunately, the symptoms of serotonin syndrome frequently begin within hours after you start taking a new medicine or increasing the dosage of one you already use. So if you experience any of them—even relatively minor symptoms, such as shivering and goose bumps, muscle twitches and/or restlessness—contact your doctor immediately. If your symptoms are mild and you catch them quickly, all you will probably need to do is stop taking the medicine that appears to be causing the problem—or one of the medicines, if you are taking two or more. Yes, more-serious serotonin syndrome can require hospital observation or admission, but much of the time, medication changes are all that is needed. In fact, symptoms can disappear within 24 hours if you stop taking whatever is causing the serotonin over-load—and, sometimes, if you also take a medicine that blocks further serotonin production within the body, such as *cyproheptadine*.

If you *do* need to do more than stop using a medi-cine or reduce its dose, there are a number of effective treatments available. Always consult your doctor about this! These treatments are used when symptoms are more severe or when serotonin syndrome is caused by antidepressants that remain in the body for a long time. Muscle relaxants are used for agitation and seizures—diazepam, best known as Valium®, and lorazepam, sold as Ativan®, are com-monly given. In some cases, when the body's oxygen levels are deplet-ed, an oxygen mask may be used. Intravenous fluids may be given for high fe-ver and dehydration, and various drugs can be given to raise or lower blood pressure and to control heart rate.

> The symptoms of serotonin syndrome frequently begin within hours after you start taking a new medicine or increasing the dosage of one you already use.

A Powerful Hormone

WHAT THE POTENTIAL serious effects of serotonin syndrome and serotonin deprivation show is simply how powerful this healing hormone is, and how important it is to keep your body in balance so that serotonin and the other healing hormones can help provide corrective balance to the stress-response hormones whose levels are constantly being raised by the pressures and difficulties of everyday modern life.

In fact, although serotonin is best known for its effects on relaxation and sleep, there is much more that it does. Its mood-regulating effects protect us against clinical depression and impulse-control disorders. It reduces feelings of hostility—again, part of its mood regulation—in ways that significantly benefit the cardiovascular system, reducing the risk of heart attack and stroke and increasing the likelihood of survival if a heart attack does occur.

And serotonin also improves social life, making it easier to develop a supportive social network—which in turn lowers your risk of everything from heart disease to mental-health problems. The way serotonin does this is by leavening negative experiences so you have a more positive

> *Serotonin can facilitate social life.*

mood and behave in a more outgoing, friendly way. This in turn improves social life—and the benefits that come with it.

Really, the best way to increase serotonin levels is through what you eat, and this is easy to do by consuming tryptophan-rich foods—not only turkey and chicken but also fish, cheese, eggs, beans, nuts and other protein-packed foods. Tryptophan is most easily converted to serotonin when you eat protein with a small amount of carbohydrates, such as legumes or brown rice. All vegetables contain carbohydrates, too—a fact often ignored in discussing dietary balance—but the amount varies widely. Ones with high water content, such as radishes and zucchini, contain the least carbohydrates; sugary ones such as tomatoes and carrots contain more; and starchy ones such as corn and sweet potatoes contain the most.

Taking Supplements

AND WHAT ABOUT supplements? In our quick-fix society, taking supplements is always tempting, but there is no such thing as a serotonin supplement. There is, however, a supplement called *5-Hydroxytryptophan* or simply 5-HTP, which is a serotonin precursor—notice the word "tryptophan" in its chemical name—and which is available over the counter. 5-HTP is usually extracted from the seeds of a shrub called *Griffonia simplicifolia*. 5-HTP is marketed as an antidepressant, sleep aid and appetite suppressant. Yes, taking it can boost serotonin levels. It induces the body to produce more of this healing hormone.

Because 5-HTP does this, various herbs relating to it are sometimes taken as supplements as well. For instance, rhodiola root—also called golden root—seems to allow more 5-HTP to enter the brain for conversion to serotonin. Kanna root, marketed as a depression treatment, contains an alkaloid called *mesembrine* that some research has shown to be a sort of natural serotonin-reuptake inhibitor. Century plant—also called sore-eye flower or poison bulb—contains substances that slow the deactivation of serotonin, so what the body produces remains active longer; and although its bulb is indeed poisonous, the supplement is not made from the bulb.

But because serotonin production is so easy to raise through dietary methods—not even requiring major changes in food consumption for most people—this is one healing hormone for which supplementation has

> The best way to increase serotonin levels is through what you eat, and this is easy to do by consuming tryptophan-rich foods.

very little justification. In fact, since eating itself is pleasurable if you take the time to enjoy your food, you can get a double benefit from consuming foods that boost serotonin production. The feeling of enjoyment itself stimulates the production of dopamine! So enjoy foods in the first place and then enjoy the effects they produce as your serotonin levels rise.

9:

The Cuddle Chemical

O F ALL THE HEALING HORMONES, the one for which the most grandiose claims have been made, the one deemed the most positive for human relationships and even for society as a whole, is oxytocin. Long receiving relatively little attention as a "female" hormone of limited and specific importance, oxytocin has in recent years seen a pendulum swing to the point that it has been considered *the* hormone to which everyone should pay far more attention—for reasons both personal and societal.

Oxytocin's name comes from two Greek words meaning "quick birth," because it is well-known for its uterine-contracting properties, discovered early in the 20th century. It is found in virtually all vertebrates and is important in stimulating milk production for breast-feeding. In fact, oxytocin was the very first polypeptide—that is, a substance made up of many molecules of amino acids—to be synthesized.

Promotes Bonding

OXYTOCIN PRODUCES AND ENHANCES feelings of contentment, calm and security, particularly around one's mate, and it reduces anxiety, lowers fear levels and significantly raises the feeling of bonding. And, importantly, it does this for *both* genders, not only for women, despite being primarily known for its effects on females.

During childbirth, oxytocin causes the uterine contractions that bring labor to its climax. After babies are
born, it is oxytocin that causes milk to be let down to
the nipples, causing two responses with which breast-
feeding mothers are familiar: contented relaxation, on
the one hand, and painful uterine contractions that
may continue for several weeks, on the other.

Stress Protection

THESE FUNCTIONS are important enough, but there is
much, much more to oxytocin than this. Its calming effect
means oxytocin is a major natural protector against the
fight-or-flight response. It appears to inhibit brain regions
associated with fear and anxiety—and seems, because it
suppresses activity in those regions, to make it possible for
orgasm to occur in both men and women, or at least to
be partially responsible for the intensity of feeling during
orgasm and the release into contentment afterwards.

Oxytocin has significant effects on *social* intercourse
as well as sexual: by suppressing fear and increasing trust,
it contributes to heightened social interactions such as
generosity, empathy and sensitivity to positive social cues.

This last finding, about oxytocin's social effects, is
fascinating, and is one key to the overall fascination with
this healing hormone. People given oxytocin in connection with an investment game, for example, were much
more likely to trust other participants than people in a
control group—but they did not display this added trust
when told they were interacting
with a computer. So oxytocin
did not make them more risk-
averse—it made them more
cooperative and empathetic.

> Oxytocin is a
> major natural
> protector against
> the fight-or-flight
> response.

Soothes Fear

OXYTOCIN DOES NOT just affect social interaction in us humans—as evidenced by an intriguing study in rats. Previous rodent studies had shown that oxytocin reduces fear response. This one went further. Research-ers were investigating how and why rats sniff each other, and found that sniffing different parts of the body means different things in rat communication. Mutual sniffing of the face typically led the less-dominant rat to back off and reduce its own sniffing—while larger, more-aggressive rats kept sniffing the subordinate's face at the same level or even increased the behavior, and would become aggressive if a subordinate did not cut back on facial sniffing. This happened consistently—*unless the domi-nant rats were given oxytocin.* In *that* case, the sniffing displays and aggression simply vanished.

> O*xytocin is a very complicated healing hormone.*

So here is the solution to war: bombard everyone on both sides with oxytocin! Somebody may actually try that, or something along those lines, sometime—maybe on a lesser scale, to control aggressive behavior in prisoners, for example—but unfortunately, on a large scale involving overt hostility, oxytocin boosting won't work. First, though, we should examine what oxytocin *can* and *does* do.

Many Sources

OXYTOCIN is a very complicated healing hormone in a lot of ways, including how the body produces it. Like other healing hormones, oxytocin is made in the brain—specifically in the *hypothalamus,* from which it is stored in the posterior lobe of the pituitary gland and then released from the gland into the blood. But that is not all: oxytocin is also produced elsewhere in the brain and in other parts of the body, including such apparently unrelated areas as the retina, the thymus, the pancreas and (less surprisingly) the placenta. Why? This is one of the mysteries of oxytocin: it is clearly important to many biological processes beyond childbirth and lactation, but to what extent and in what way is not clear.

Taking Supplements

UNLIKE several other healing hormones, oxytocin *can* be taken directly, in supplement form. In fact, it is sold by prescription under the names Pitocin® and Syntocinon®. But oxytocin supplementation is not a matter of taking a pill: the hormone is destroyed in the gastrointestinal tract, so it must be given by injection or as a nasal spray—as we saw in the relationship anecdotes at the start of this book.

The second of those methods, nasal spray, is not much of an inconvenience, so experiments with oxytocin are relatively easy to do, and they have proliferated. It has been tested to stimulate breastfeeding, with mixed results. It has been tried to help people who suffer from severe social anxiety and a variety of mood disorders—again, with mixed results. It has even been used to treat autism, and has been shown effective in producing more-appropriate social behavior, at least in clinical trials.

Injected oxytocin has been shown in studies of rats to have very significant sexual impact, making females more sexually receptive and giving males spontaneous erections when injected into their cerebrospinal fluid.

No, it has not been tested this way in humans, but injected oxytocin *is* used to induce labor and improve uterine tone in women with postpartum hemorrhage. And in veterinary medicine, it is commonly used to make birth easier and to stimulate milk release.

Oxytocin in Humans

BUT BACK TO USES among humans. Pair bonding, empathy, anxiety reduction, extroversion, feelings of trust—oxytocin is involved in all of these and more. And you don't have to use it nasally to get the benefits—you don't have to "use" anything at all to raise oxytocin levels. This healing hormone is unique in the way it is self-reinforcing: behaving in the various ways explained later in this chapter will cause your body to produce more oxytocin, which will cause you to be even more comfortable behaving in those ways, which will cause even more oxytocin production, and so on.

> B*ehaving in certain ways will cause your body to produce more oxytocin.*

Yes, there are limits, which are different for every person and depend on psychological factors as much as physical ones. But the important point is that this powerful healing hormone, which is involved in so many aspects of human relationships and interrelationships, is one whose levels are easy for most people to raise—and that is very good news.

Social Facilitator

GOOD NEWS for couples, anyway. What makes oxytocin easier to increase than other healing hormones is that you simply have to take advantage of the natural circumstances under which it is produced. And those circumstances relate to bonding. Think of oxytocin as a *social facilitator* and you will have a key to what it does and how to get your body to make more of it.

There needs to be some social basis to begin with, which is why the investment-game trust experiment got different results when people thought they were dealing with a computer rather than another human. By the same token, oxytocin's effects are ramped up, and the body produces more of it, when you interact with someone to whom you are already close—the hormone reinforces your feeling of being bonded. So couples have a wide variety of ways to increase their oxytocin levels and, by doing so, increase their feelings of closeness and commitment—leading to still more oxytocin production and still closer feelings, in that self-reinforcing loop that is characteristic of this healing hormone.

Oxytocin Boosters

- Display affection
- Walk holding hands or with arms linked
- Drape arms around each other
- Stop while walking for a hug or cuddle

Hugging and cuddling are good oxytocin boosters in private, too, so give yourself plenty of time to show affection in bed. Oxytocin levels rise during foreplay, leap to two or more times the normal amount at orgasm, and produce the post-coital feelings of relaxation, warmth, comfort and relaxed sleepiness. So allow plenty of time for sexual encounters. Enjoy your partner thoroughly from the start—show affection that includes sexual touching but is not limited to it. Talk about how you feel about your partner—engage all your senses, including taste, smell, sight and hearing as well as touch. Express your pleasure with your partner out loud, in sounds as well as words. Make it clear how much you are enjoying being with him or her. Allow plenty of time for sex— and for cuddling afterwards. Talk about how you feel. Thank your partner. Say how appreciative you are. Even though oxytocin causes relaxation and tends to make us fall asleep after sex, try to nuzzle into each other and fall asleep gradually and while holding each other close. The more forms of physical intimacy you create between you, the more oxytocin you will both produce.

Physical touch is not even necessary to raise oxytocin production if you are in a romantic relationship. Just *thinking* about your partner can cause your body to make more oxytocin—assuming you are thinking pleasant, happy thoughts, of course. When you find your thoughts drifting to your partner during work, allow them to drift—really think about him or her, about how much you enjoy each other's company, about how special the relationship is.

Set aside "relationship thinking time" for the express purpose of considering why this relationship is more meaningful than others you may have had. Think of what makes the relationship special and of why you feel special because of it. Think of ways in which you and your partner complement each other—things that are better because you are together—things you do better as a team than you could as individuals. The more thoughts about your partner and the relationship you come up with, the more you encourage your body to produce oxytocin.

> *Just* thinking *about your romantic partner can cause your body to make more oxytocin.*

And this remarkable at-a-distance effect opens up additional ways to boost oxytocin levels, because the body creates more of this healing hormone when you think about *anything* familiar and comforting. The effect is increased if you immerse yourself in whatever that may be, just as it is higher when you are with your romantic partner than when you are apart.

Thinking happily about a favorite comfort food can raise your oxytocin level, but actually making the food and engaging with the ingredients through touch and smell will raise oxytocin levels more. Remembering a gorgeous sunrise will raise oxytocin, but waking up early to experience one will lead to a greater increase. Recalling a performance of music you love will boost oxytocin levels, but playing a recording of the music will raise them even higher. Oxytocin is an *experiential* hormone, and while thinking about pleasurable experiences is enough to cause the body to make more of it, actually indulging in those experiences is even better.

Enjoy Eating

Try this. Choose a food that you really enjoy eating. Think about it—in detail. What makes it special? What is its taste, its texture, its "mouth feel"? What associations do you have with it that make it so pleasant? When did you first eat it? Under what circumstances? When do you usually eat it now? Is it a treat or something you try to eat regularly because you enjoy it so much?

The more you think about the food, the more you really imagine what it looks, feels and tastes like, the more you are encouraging your body to produce oxytocin. And then, for an even bigger oxytocin boost, eat some of the food! Do not gobble it, even if all your thinking has made you eager to do so.

Eat slowly and while really thinking about it. If it is, say, chocolate—a favorite food for many of us—do not just pop some in your mouth. Touch it, hold it, feel it start to melt on your fingers, think about what it is like to experience it on your skin—and when you do eat it, eat the tiniest possible bit, really savoring the flavor, the touch, the way it melts in your mouth, the way it feels as you swallow it. The idea is to immerse yourself in the eating experience—fully appreciating your special food and being fully aware of the experience involved in consuming it.

For Singles, Too

THAT OXYTOCIN is experiential is a good thing for people who are not happily pair-bonded. So much attention has been paid to oxytocin as it relates to love and intimate affection that the plight of singles has been largely neglected. But the fact that oxytocin rises in response to pleasurable experiences, and even thoughts about pleasurable experiences, means that singles too can effectively raise their oxytocin levels—and thereby increase their comfort in social situations, thus increasing the chance that they will connect with another person and end up as part of a couple. Hormones do not have "intentions," but if we imagine that they do, this would be oxytocin's: to help people get together and stay that way.

10:

Oxytocin Boosters

SOME PEOPLE are so determined to increase their bodies' oxytocin production that they go to "cuddle parties." These are non-sexual group gatherings exploring physical intimacy—a fad created in New York City in the early 2000s that quickly spread worldwide. Oxytocin supplements are sometimes used at these parties, but not necessarily, because the non-sexual, friendly, affectionate touching is itself an oxytocin booster.

Sometimes called "puppy pile parties" for the way people taking part in them resemble piles of pups squirming onto and around each other, cuddle parties received considerable media attention and a fair amount of sensational coverage—including being featured on several TV shows. For all the hype, cuddle parties do have genuine value as oxytocin boosters for people who come to them with an understanding that they are about nonsexual closeness. Here is a typical writeup by a Cuddle Party organizer:

> "You can wear your PJ's, eat snacks and tea, and meet some new fun folks. Expand your kindness quotient, connect with your compassion, and know that what you choose will be honored. Together we will create a safe space for ease of self-discovery."

If you like this idea, try going to a party! Check for ones in your area on any search engine or through social-gathering Web sites.

Cuddle Your Pet

WHEN IT COMES TO OXYTOCIN, it is particularly important not to define bonding too narrowly, because another way you can rise your oxytocin level—whether you are single or part of a couple—is with pets. The loyalty, uncritical acceptance and love of a dog, the comfort to be drawn from a purring cat, even the enjoyment of a bird on your finger or shoulder or a snake draped around your arm, can be just the thing to increase oxytocin production. The touch is what matters, coupled with the feeling of relaxation and pleasure associated with the pet. When it comes to companion animals, singles are not excluded from ways of raising oxytocin production—and of course couples with pets have additional ways of boosting this healing hormone.

Experience Your Pet

Turn off the TV, the computer, and your cell phone! Focus fully on your pet. Give your pet all your attention. Notice how you feel when you interact with it. Don't try to "get inside your pet's head." Simply enjoy being fully in your pet's presence, without distractions. Tune into your feelings about your pet. Think about what gives you pleasure about your relationship with this pet, which things you find entrancing, amusing, silly.

The idea is to be-
come more aware of your
feelings toward your
pet—and your feelings

> Touch is what matters,
> coupled with the feeling
> of relaxation and pleasure.

that your pet inspires or reminds you about, such as
love, loyalty and attachment. It is through this "feeling
connection" that your body raises your oxytocin level.

Give Hugs; Get Hugs

GIVE HUGS WITH ENTHUSIASM—and often. Hug your
friends, not just your partner. Hug your kids frequently.
Hug other people's kids, too. Ask first! Remember the
pet exercise? Hug your pet! That may not work with a
fish, but it is great with a dog, cat, hamster, ferret, and
even with reptiles, which love the warmth of your body
and are happy being held and hugged. (BTW, even
snakes hug back!)

The more hugs you give, the more hugging gives
back to you in the form of higher oxytocin production.
And *get* lots of hugs, too—make it clear that you enjoy
being hugged, and encourage people to hug you back.
Some people think they need a reason to hug, but hugging itself is the reason! Use it often!

Touch Your Child

THE CLOSENESS OF A CHILD in your lap is an un-
matched way of boosting oxytocin. Read regularly to
your child—even those who are too young to understand stories will enjoy pictures and the sound of your
voice. Set aside time every day to read with your child,
or do other activities that will keep him or her in your
lap—yes, even watching TV is better if the two of you
are physically close.

For babies, get a sling that lets you carry your little one in front of you and stay close all the time you are walking—it is like a permanent hug appliance! Babies readily and peacefully fall asleep in slings, lulled by the closeness of the adult carrying them and the rhythmic nature of walking. When not using the sling, have plenty of floor time with a baby—being face to face, looking into his or her eyes and responding to baby's movements and discovery of the world.

Rock together in a rocking chair sometimes—the rhythmic motion lulls both of you and is tremendously relaxing. All forms of physical contact with babies and children can be wonderful oxytocin boosters. Apply lotion or oil to baby and really focus on feeling that wonderful baby skin—gently brush a baby's or child's hair and marvel at the hair's thickness or thinness, the way it grows, its color, its smell.

All these experiences are strong bonding ones, and all are excellent ways to raise your oxytocin level—and your child's. And do not think oxytocin-boosting bonding has to end as children grow. Play wrestling with kids can be a lot of fun, and the close physical contact works well into the preteen years. And for older preteens and teenagers, something as simple as a pat on the back and an affectionate touch of the shoulder when you walk past can do a lot to soothe the increasing angst of later childhood—calling oxytocin into play for both you and your child to increase the bond between you.

Dance with a Friend

YOU DON'T HAVE TO BE Fred Astaire or Ginger Rogers to get an oxytocin "hit" from ballroom dancing. Old favorites like tango, the swing, the waltz, or salsa,

require partners and touching and a genuine partner-
ship in motion, with each of you paying close attention
to the other's body positions and responding to them.
Synchronizing yourselves
this way actually brings
you into harmony, all the
more so since the music

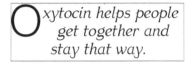

O*xytocin helps people
get together and
stay that way.*

playing is harmonious. All that harmonization is great
for oxytocin levels.

Book Clubs

A GREAT WAY to meet and interact with others. Simply sharing thoughts and interests with other people
can help raise your oxytocin level—you are close not
only physically, as you sit around a table or in a circle,
but also mentally, as you discuss shared experience and
comment on it.

Learn a Skill

LEARNING A SKILL, such as a foreign language, is a solo
activity in that you need to learn to speak and write
on your own. But when done in a group of learners,
it brings people together in a supportive environment
toward a common goal—the fact that everyone will
reach the goal in his or her own time and in a different way becomes irrelevant, and the supportiveness
helps everyone move toward the shared goal and boosts
oxytocin as well.

Because oxytocin is a hormone of connection,
nearly all the attention paid to it involves becoming
more strongly attached—whether to people, pets, foods
or experiences. This is no surprise. But oxytocin *does*
have some surprises in store.

Stress Buffer

THE BONDING ELEMENT of oxytocin does, it turns out, help you in some unexpected ways. It turns out that oxytocin is not only released in higher amounts when people are relaxed, comfortable and in bonding relationships. The body also produces it under exactly the opposite circumstance, when people are subjected to social separation and the stress that comes with it. You would expect stress of this sort to result in heightened production of the fight-or-flight hormone *cortisol*, and this does occur. But, surprisingly, oxytocin production rises as well. One study found that women with less-positive partner relationships and more difficulty in their social connections actually had higher levels of both oxytocin and cortisol in their bodies than did women in better relationships.

In other words, when we are comfortable and feeling attached, oxytocin levels rise to preserve and enhance our connections. But when we have stress responses to social circumstances, this healing hormone rises to make us more amenable to social connections that will lead to stress reduction.

So what do we do with all this information showing that rather than being a "cuddle hormone" or "love hormone," oxytocin is a hormone of nuance? Natural increases in oxytocin levels certainly do have demonstrable benefits in countering the stress response, improving social relationships, increasing bonding, and leading to a greater feeling of "connectedness." And in light of the fact that the body produces oxytocin both when we are comfortable, connected and bonded and when we are feeling distanced and dislocated, we can rely on oxytocin to help us develop bonds and cement the ones we already have.

This means that the many techniques for raising levels of this healing hormone should become part of your daily routine at *all* times in your life. Look back at the many possibilities for boosting oxytocin levels that we have discussed, from expressions of affection toward your partner and children to focused interaction with pets and even taking dance classes. What you can do for yourself on an ongoing basis is to practice ways of increasing oxytocin in your everyday life—helping to counter the stressors that are always there. Instead of looking to boost oxytocin only occasionally or under certain circumstances, incorporate oxytocin-raising routines into your daily schedule.

Like the other healing hormones, oxytocin provides a natural way for your body's internal mechanisms to counteract many of the external stressors and pressures that could otherwise become overwhelming.

11:

Stress Talk

WE RESPOND EMOTIONALLY to words. We all know that, and so do advertisers and propagandists. By changing the words we say to ourselves—our self-talk—we can change the way we respond.

We Stress Ourselves

WE TEND TO THINK OF WORDS as reflecting reality, and when it comes to factual statements, they do: "It is raining." "That building is four stories tall." "The dog is barking." But unthinking acceptance of words as "reality reflectors" gets us into trouble when we are dealing with *subjective* experience—with our feelings about events in our lives. In that case, words *shape* reality. "I'll never get this project finished." "I don't have time to exercise." "This heavy traffic is awful. It'll be a disaster if I miss my flight."

Objectively, it is unlikely that the project will *never* be finished. As for time to exercise, you know very well that you can find 10 or 15 minutes a day for something you really want to do, like watching your favorite TV show. And traffic? Yes, it *may* make you miss your flight, but that isn't a disaster. A plane crash is a disaster—missing your flight is an inconvenience. Each of these remarks is an overstatement that *shapes* reality by making things seem worse than they actually are. These overstatements redefine common life events into *threats*.

There is a part of our minds that is constantly alert for threats. Most of the time, we are unaware of this part of ourselves—our Vigilant Self. We humans are, after all, rather vulnerable. We don't have claws and big teeth and thick skin with rough fur, as grizzly bears do. So for creatures as ill-equipped for physical combat as we are, forewarned is forearmed. The sooner you become aware of a threat, the more likely you can deal with it, including fleeing—getting out of there.

Your Vigilant Self operates in an all-or-nothing manner—there are no gradations of threat. The Vigilant Self is constantly asking: "Is there a threat? Or am I safe?" When the answer is "there's a threat," the Vigilant Self sounds the alarm, triggering the stress response that turns on the sympathetic nervous system's fight-or-flight response, flooding our bodies with stress hormones.

Self-Talk

WE ARE CONSTANTLY THINKING—talking to ourselves—telling ourselves the meaning of things going on around us. "That's Sally. She's pretty." "That's Jack. He's nice because he gave me tomatoes." Psychologists call this "self-talk," and it is powerful. We talk to ourselves nonstop all day.

And it is amazing how we constantly stress ourselves without realizing we are doing it with our own thinking—our self-talk. We tell ourselves that a red light that holds us up for two or three minutes is a calamity that will cause dire things to happen. We tell ourselves that a curt word or criticism from the boss means she is giving us a bad performance review. We tell ourselves that falling behind on one credit-card payment means we are about to go bankrupt. These are all extreme, exaggerated pictures of events around us that keep us in a state of constant upset and stress.

Objectively, none of this is true; and when we can look objectively at the situations, we *know* the awful consequences are highly unlikely. But your body reacts viscerally instead of with objectivity, which triggers the stress response. Yet it doesn't have to be that way.

When we talk to ourselves in negative, stress-provoking ways, we listen with EARs rather than our rational mind. EAR is an acronym for Event/Appraisal/Response, and it is a convenient way to think about how self-talk induces the fight-or-flight response. The Event is the objective, real-world occurrence, such as a traffic jam or a negative remark from the boss. The Appraisal is how we appraise the situation—what we tell ourselves *about* the significance of the event. And the Response is our reaction, which is *not* to the Event but to the Appraisal—what we tell ourselves *about* the event.

Thinking with EARs

E — Event: Boss makes curt remark.

A — Appraisal: She's against me and is going to give me a poor review.

R — Response: Anger, anxiety, insomnia.

Understanding EARs reveals that we are not helpless victims of circumstances, but we are creating our own "reality." And that means that by changing the way you talk to yourself about events in your life, you can manage and reduce the stress you feel. You cannot alter the events themselves, but you *can* alter the way you talk to yourself about those events *and thereby alter your response*. For example, instead of telling yourself that the boss is out to get you and is going to give you a bad review, you could tell yourself that the boss is in a bad mood because of problems at home.

> **E** — Event: Boss makes curt remark.
>
> **A** — Appraisal: She is stressed out over problems at home.
>
> **R** — Response: Understanding, sympathy, forgiveness.

Gaining Control

WHEN A NEGATIVE or unpleasant event happens, we tend to think that something is happening *to* us, and this makes us feel helpless. Since we humans are so physically vulnerable, lacking those claws and big teeth, feeling helpless is a serious fight-or-flight activator. Feelings of helplessness and the corollary of feeling put-upon—"how can they do this to me?"—signal "threat" to our Vigilant Self and trigger the release of a cascade of stress hormones, not because of the events that occur but because of how we talk to ourselves *about* those events.

People can respond very differently to identical situations as a result of how they think about those situations. For example, someone who is afraid of snakes will experience stress and a fight-or-flight response upon seeing a snake in the path.

> **E** — Event: A snake is in the path.
>
> **A** — Appraisal: Oh no! It's going to bite me! I'll be poisoned and die!
>
> **R** — Response: Fear, panic, screaming, attempt to escape.

By comparison, a person with experience with the reptiles, such as a herpetologist, is more likely simply to observe the snake with interest and possibly even pick it up. Same circumstances, different reactions—one resulting in stress, one not, and all because of EARs.

E — Event: A snake is in the path.

A — Appraisal: Oh wow! Look at that beautiful snake. I love snakes. They are so interesting.

R — Response: Pleasure, curiosity, picking up the snake.

The good thing about understanding EARs is that it gives us a powerful way to manage and reduce stress. You do not have to change what happens, which is impossible—just change the way you talk to yourself *about* events to reduce stress. And that *is* possible.

12:

Reword Self-Talk

WE CAN SOOTHE WITH WORDS, or we can incite fear and anger with words, or we can soothe ourselves by changing what we say to ourselves—changing our words.

The first step in doing this is to become aware of the things you tell yourself about events in your life. When you catch yourself getting stressed, notice what you were thinking as the stress came on. For example, suppose you are ordering lunch at a fast-food place and notice tension coming on. If you listen to what you are saying to yourself, you might hear, "I should order something healthful," as you look at the menu.

Or suppose you feel anger welling up when your wife calls to say she will be working late and for you to go without her to the movie you had planned to see together that evening. If you catch yourself, you may hear, "She promised and she *should* keep her promises. She's so inconsiderate—and mean!" If you talk to yourself like that, no wonder you react with anger, or maybe disappointment or depression—all of those being stressful.

> *By changing shoulds to preferences you can change how you respond to events.*

Notice What You Tell Yourself

STOP READING. Put this book down and bring to mind a
time when you—or another—should have done something and didn't. Recall a relatively inconsequential,
but annoying, situation; don't use a major disappointment for this experiment. Bring the event to mind and
relive it for several seconds. Don't try to change it;
instead, let it run for a while until you begin feeling the
emotions you felt during the real event.

What are those emotions? Annoyance? Disappointment? Tension? Anger? Fear? Foreboding? Loneliness?
Confusion? Now, turn the dial back a little to notice
what you were thinking—*what you were telling yourself*—
about the event as you lived through it. It may take some
practice to capture this self-talk, but when you do, you'll
probably discover implied or actual *shoulds*, *oughts*, and
musts—unfulfilled demands and obligations.

Many of us feel as if things happen "to" us. We are
victims, helplessly swept away in the flood of happen-
ings. Actually, we create this perception with our self-
talk. An event happens: your spouse cancels a date for
the movie you wanted to see. You appraise or interpret
the situation: she should keep promises. You evaluate:
she is mean and inconsiderate. And then you react to
the appraisal—what you told yourself about the situation. And so you get angry.

We all do this. This process is what mystics are
referring to when they say that "we create our own reality." Recalling EARs, we talk ourselves into interpreta-
tions of situations that can be totally wrong and "out
there," which we take as "real" and then respond to
with stress when we believe something to be threatening—which is a great deal of the time.

"Shoulding" Yourself

IF YOU'RE LIKE MOST OF US, you probably worry about what you and others "should" do, which can be called "shoulding yourself." We easily fall into the trap of thinking about what "ought" to happen and what "should" be done. By shoulding, you are dwelling on how you or another person are doing it—whatever "it" is—all wrong and failing to meet expectations. This triggers all kinds of worries, fears and anger, especially when the other person is not acting as he or she should. When something does not happen as it "should," we tend to view it as awful and tell ourselves we just cannot stand it, that it is terrible and a disaster. Our reactive minds read this as a threat— and the stress response kicks in.

Consider this. Suppose your daughter is late and doesn't call. You may think to yourself, "My daughter should call when she is late. She was late but didn't call—and that is wrong, bad, awful." Perhaps you view her failure to call as insubordination, a rebellion (threat) against your authority. Or perhaps you worry that she could be injured or worse—how would you know if she didn't call to explain her tardiness?

> Many of us feel like victims, swept away in the flood of happenings.

The good news is that you can change reality by changing the way you talk to yourself about events in your life. The rule of thumb is to change shoulds to preferences.

Steps to Take

HERE IS HOW IT WORKS. The first step is to catch yourself shoulding. You can do this by recalling events, as
you did in the above exercise, and catching yourself
in the moment. If you catch yourself shoulding, don't
try to change anything. Instead, listen to yourself and
watch what happens. The more objective you can be in
your observation, the better.

One way is to imagine you are a scientist observing
your subject—you. Don't try to change; just watch and
listen to the self-talk. As soon as you have a chance,
write the self-talk down. You might carry a few index
cards in your pocket for "recording your data." When
you have gathered several "should" thoughts, write
them in a list on the left side of a piece of paper. At the
top of the list, write "Shoulds."

Now thoughtfully brainstorm a new statement that
is a preference and not a demand. This may seem a
little artificial at first, but that's because it is a different
way of thinking, using a different set of words. For the
example of your spouse working late and missing the
movie, you might write: "I prefer that my wife keep her
promises." And secondly, "I'd rather go to the movie
with my wife than alone."

Preference Flashcards

LEARNING IS MORE FUN when it's a game, and that
includes learning to change the way you talk to yourself. After you capture a few dozen shoulds, which you
thoughtfully rewrite as preferences, get out a pack of
index cards. Write a should on one side of a card; then
write the corresponding preference on the other side.
For example, you might write, "My daughter should

call when she is late!" on the should side; then write "I prefer that my daughter call when she is late" on the preference side of the card. Repeat this with all of the shoulds you have transformed to preferences.

Rewrite Shoulds as Preferences

My daughter should call when she will be home late.	I prefer that my daughter call when she will be home late.
My spouse ought to make more money.	I would like my spouse to make more money.
I'm such a pig. I should exercise more.	I would like to exercise more and to get into better shape.
Everyone should like me.	I prefer that everyone like me.

You now have a set of Should to Preference flashcards. Read one of the shoulds, then convert it to a preference. Flip the card to compare your answer with the preference on the card. This will seem deceptively easy. But just as when you were a kid and did multiplication-table drills so knowing the answers would become "rote," that is what you want here: to overwrite the bad shoulding habit with a preference habit. And in the beginning, it is helpful if this is rote—automatic— because whether you realize it or not, your shoulding is automatic.

Practice Underreacting

WE REACT TO THE WORLD AROUND US all the time— or rather to the world that we think is around us. We do this by creating reactive statements that we say to

ourselves, usually unconsciously. A bad traffic jam as we
head to work may lead us to tell ourselves, "I'm going
to be late for that big meeting and lose my job!" We are
not really reacting to the traffic—we are imagining that
the traffic will create a situation that will cause a calamity for us, and our self-talk becomes a highly negative
reactive statement.

More to the point, this is an over-reactive statement—because what is really the chance that being
late for a single meeting will cost us our job? Reactive
statements are the way we constantly respond to what
we perceive in the world—which means that changing
reactive statements can have a big impact on our feelings of stress. The idea is to go from over-reactive statements, which heighten our feeling of being threatened
and therefore engage the sympathetic nervous system,
to under-reactive ones.

Under-reactive statements short-circuit the sympathetic nervous system's response to a crisis by showing
that what is happening is not a crisis—not a threat.
This prevents the flooding of stress hormones. Interest-
ingly, we all know—intellectually—that we do better in
a real crisis by staying calm than by panicking. But in
the many pseudo-crises of everyday life—a traffic jam,
the arrival of an unexpectedly large credit-card bill, a
power outage—many of us overreact, telling ourselves,
"This is a disaster!" This results in a surge of stress hormones, throwing our body out of balance and making it
harder to come up with a solution to whatever is con-
fronting us.

Let's take a look at some under-reactive statements
that we can use to push back against the tendency to
see every objectively minor setback of modern life as a
tragedy.

Under-Reactive Statements

- This is not a big deal.
- This will pass.
- This is only anxiety.
- Ten years from now I won't remember this.
- It just doesn't matter.
- This isn't an emergency.
- I'm not in a hurry.
- This is not worth getting upset over.
- It's only money.
- So what?

When you are calm and not in what seems like a crisis situation, practice coming up with under-reactive statements until you have a good stock of them in your mind. Write them down, too—this will help cement them into your memory. Be sure to do this while you are feeling calm and not threatened or pressured, because you need to make the under-reactive statements an integral part of your self-talk so you can call on them the next time you do find yourself in a stressful situation.

Once you have a good sense of under-reactive statements and a good collection of them, try applying them to situations in your life that you know usually cause you to feel stressed. You can write down the sort of self-talk in which you know you engage on the left side of a piece of paper—and then, on the right side, write down an under-reactive statement that will help you stay calm to avoid the stress response, the next time you encounter the situation in the real world.

Reactive to Under-Reactive Statements

Being stuck in traffic is awful!	I'd rather not be stuck in this traffic.
This pouring rain is horrific for driving!	What a downpour! I'll drive with extra caution.
The company's new strategy is a disaster.	I can handle change and confusion.
Being stuck on hold is awful!	I don't like being on hold but it does give me a chance to relax.
Her politics are infuriating.	I can listen to views I don't agree with.
My wife's overspending is bankrupting us!	My wife's spending needs correction.
Oh no! I'm having an asthma attack. How will I give my presentation?!	My chest is getting tight. I'll grab some asthma medicine at the drugstore on the way to the meeting.

There are many ways to avoid over-reactive words and change them to under-reactive ones. You already know how to do this and probably do it often—without necessarily realizing it. For example, if your boss makes a reorganization proposal that seems completely wrong-headed to you, you know not to blurt out, "That's the stupidest idea I've ever heard." Even if you momentarily think that, you will not say it. You will say something like, "I'm not sure that will work." If you are having trouble keeping up with bills and your wife says she really wants a new car, you may think something like, "Are you out of your mind?" But you will not say that if you want to maintain your relationship. You will say something such as, "We really can't afford that now—let's pay down our credit cards first." And you may add, "And let's figure out how we can budget ourselves so we can buy a car soon."

These are examples of two effective techniques for avoiding overreaction. One is using milder words, changing "stupidest idea" to "I'm not sure that will work" and giving a reasonable rather than angry, stress-filled response to the new-car suggestion. The other is changing negatives to positives, suggesting a budget that will make car buying possible instead of harping on the idea that the whole notion is out of the question. Try to apply these techniques to your daily self-talk about everyday frustrations and irritations.

Change Can Be Slow

DON'T EXPECT rewording your self-talk to take hold in your mind immediately. It takes vigilance and practice to make any change, especially when habits are entrenched. It takes practice to become aware of your negative self-statements and your awfulizing of circumstances and how it sets off the stress response. The way we talk to ourselves is deeply ingrained, maybe even learned very early from our parents. If you are 30 years old, think of how many days, months and years you have been practicing saying negative things to yourself.

Don't expect to come up with preferences and under-reactive statements on the spot, especially when thinking about something that "really matters." This is why it is easier—and more likely to be effective—when you write down the should-statement or the reactive-statement and then write down a translation to a preference or an under-reactive statement. Practice changing shoulds to preferences and reactive statements to under-reactive statements when you are calm and feeling relaxed.

Creating flashcards to drill yourself or even simply reading the translations over and over will help. The new words and ways of saying things to yourself need to be readily accessible—on the tip of your tongue—to be effective. Don't wait until you are stressing to try to use new words in your self-talk. You'll just fall back to old self-talk habits—and be very discouraged. It takes about a month to create a new habit—longer if the old habit you are trying to replace is one you have held onto for a very long time. Patterns of negative or positive self-talk are often deeply ingrained, dating back to childhood. The good news is that you can start changing them anytime—using your mind to relieve stress and allow your healing hormones to flow more freely. You just need to allow yourself enough time for the new, less-reactive, lower-stress pattern to displace the old one.

Praise Yourself

HIDDEN IN THE USE OF SHOULDS and over-reactive words is a focus on negatives and on the ways that we are failing. This keeps us trapped in bad habits. Habits are hard to break—and can be next to impossible to change when we focus on how we are doing something all wrong. It is important to notice and acknowledge small steps to change. Talk to yourself in positive, self-supportive, rewarding ways. This will help you to change your stressful self-talk.

When you practice, notice how you are able to make the transformation—and praise yourself for doing so. For example, tell yourself, "I can do this. I can change my thinking habits." Or you might say, "Good. Got that one." Or "Hey, I'm good at this."

Gaining Control

BY REWRITING THE WORDS that you use to describe events, you gain a sense of control over your reaction to those events. This will promote your health, psychologically and physically. Overall psychological stress is closely related to disease. Remember that, given the opportunity, your body will produce more healing hormones and will damp down the stress response that can be so debilitating. If there is a single underlying idea that unites de-stressing with healing hormones, it is to let your body do what it does best—return to a sense of balance, of homeostasis, that translates into an overall feeling of well-being. This is by no means always a simple thing to accomplish, but you can do it—and when you do, you will experience a remarkable resurgence of healing hormones that will help you realize that you *can* cope with all the difficulties that life throws at you.

13:

Testosterone & Estrogen

THE HUMAN BODY PRODUCES more than 50 hormones, which come in three classifications: eicosanoid, peptide and steroid. None of them comes with a neat label such as "fight-or-flight" or "healing." We make those labels up ourselves so as to make sense, with our conscious mind, of what the body does on an entirely unconscious, autonomic level. Recall that the sympathetic and parasympathetic nervous systems have near-opposite purposes—excitation and calm, respectively—and use specific hormones to fulfill their responsibility to promote homeostasis except in times of a perceived direct threat. Cortisol, epinephrine and norepinephrine are the primary components of the fight-or-flight response, while the substances we are calling healing hormones—nitric oxide, dopamine, endorphins, serotonin and oxytocin—are the primary relaxants and "stress busters."

> *Many hormones have attracted public and scientific attention, including some that have become popular as supplements.*

There are many other hormones that have attracted public and scientific attention, including some that have become popular as supplements and have been widely touted in the mass media and on the Internet. Indeed, some people would consider *these* to be healing hormones for their ability to counteract certain specific mental and physical issues. You have almost certainly heard of these hormones and heard many claims for them. Let's take a look at the realities.

Testosterone

TESTOSTERONE IS A HORMONE produced primarily in the testicles and important because it helps maintain many elements of men's health, sexual and otherwise. Proper testosterone production is essential to maintain men's bone density, manage the body's fat distribution, and maintain muscle strength and mass. Testosterone is important to the blood as well, affecting the production of red blood cells. These are all in addition to testosterone's well-known importance in keeping a man's sex drive going and his sperm production sufficient for reproduction.

Less well known is the fact that women as well as men produce testosterone—women's ovaries make it—and it is important for women's bodies as well as men's. Men tend to worry about whether they produce too little testosterone. But for women, a greater concern is often the production of too much. If you are a woman whose body produces too much testosterone, you may have irregular menstrual periods—or none. You may have more body hair than the average woman, and possibly frontal balding. And you may have acne, an enlarged clitoris, increased muscle mass, and a deep voice.

It is less well known that women also produce testosterone.

Nevertheless, testosterone is primarily important to men—comparable to estrogen in women, as we will see. A man's testosterone levels peak during adolescence and early adulthood. As men get older, their testoster-

one level gradually drops—typically about one percent
per year after age 30. By later life, men tend to develop
a variety of signs that we usually think of as "typical of aging" and that are actually caused by reduced
testosterone levels. The one with which most people
are familiar is changes in sexual function. As a man's
testosterone level drops, he may experience an overall
reduction in sexual desire, may have fewer spontaneous
erections—such as typically occur during sleep—and
may become infertile.

Other Effects

LESS WELL KNOWN, although equally important for an
aging man's health, reduced testosterone can produce
changes in sleep patterns, including insomnia and other
sleep disturbances. A man's entire body shape and
appearance can be affected as testosterone levels fall:
body fat increases, muscle bulk and strength decrease,
and bone density drops, making men more vulnerable to fractures if they fall. Low testosterone can also
cause men to develop swollen or tender breasts, lose
hair, and experience hot flashes similar to the ones that
many women complain of during menopause. A man
whose testosterone level has fallen will tend to have
less energy than he did when his testosterone levels
were high—and this can lead to a variety of emotional
effects, including decreased motivation and self-confi-
dence, sadness or depression, and trouble concentrating
or remembering things.

No one wants any of these symptoms, and if testosterone therapy will head them off or reverse them,
many men will jump at it—and have. But it is important to understand that these signs are frequently
a normal part of aging. When that is not the case,

the symptoms may still not be caused by low testosterone—they could result from various underlying factors,
such as medication side effects, thyroid problems, clinical
depression or excessive alcohol use. The only way to find
out with certainty if you have low testosterone is with a
blood test—and even that test will not show for sure that
reduced testosterone levels
have *caused* the symptoms.

> A *blood test is the only way to find out with certainty if you have low testosterone.*

Still, testosterone *can*
be responsible for many
of these undesirable age-
related effects, and this
explains why many men regard testosterone as a healing
hormone and are eager to try it. In theory, testosterone
supplements can increase muscle mass, sharpen memory
and concentration, boost libido, and improve energy
level. Testosterone sounds like the ultimate anti-aging
formula.

Remember, though, that your body tends to stay in
balance—homeostasis—and that this is true throughout
life, even though the specifics of the balance change
over time. The health benefits of testosterone therapy
for age-related testosterone decline are not, it turns out,
clear for most people—although they *are* clear for *some.*

Hypogonadism

IN A DISEASE called hypogonadism, the body cannot produce normal amounts of testosterone because of a problem
with the testicles or with the pituitary gland—which,
among other functions, controls the testicles. For men
with hypogonadism, testosterone replacement therapy can
improve the symptoms of low testosterone. But for men
whose testosterone decline is simply age-related and not
disease-related, the picture is much less clear.

Remember that the body will accept only so much supplementation—for example, if you take vitamins to help your body boost production of healing hormones, taking *more* vitamins will not lead to *more* hormone production; above a certain level, your body will simply excrete the vitamins. Similarly, testosterone supplementation in otherwise healthy men does not restore memory, muscle mass and sex drive—although for men who *believe* it will do this, there may be some improvements because of the placebo effect, in which the body itself makes changes because we are convinced that it will change!

It is simply unclear whether testosterone therapy has any real benefit for older men who are otherwise healthy. Few scientifically valid studies have looked at the use of testosterone therapy in men who have testosterone levels that are normal for their age—and some research has had mixed and surprising results. For example, in one study, healthy men who took testosterone medications did have increased muscle mass—but they did not gain any strength.

Risks of Testosterone Therapy

TESTOSTERONE therapy also carries risks, which men who are eager to try it should not ignore. It may contribute to sleep apnea—a potentially serious disorder in which breathing repeatedly stops and starts during sleep. Because testosterone is associated with maintenance and production of red blood cells, testosterone therapy can cause the body to make *too many* of these cells, resulting in a condition called *polycythemia*—which can increase the risk of heart disease.

Testosterone may also cause

It is unclear whether testosterone therapy has any real benefit for older men who are otherwise healthy.

acne or other skin reactions, and it can cause noncancerous growth of the prostate, known as *benign prostatic hyperplasia*. In men who already have prostate cancer, it may stimulate the cancer's growth. It can also cause men to develop enlarged breasts. And while natural testosterone levels are important for fertility, testosterone therapy may reduce sperm production or cause testicles to shrink.

What About Supplements?

DESPITE THE RISKS, it is certainly tempting for men who are feeling the effects of aging to try testosterone therapy—and this is a hormone that *can* be directly supplemented. In fact, when doctors prescribe it for treatment of hypogonadism, they may have patients use it as injections, pellets, patches or gels; all these methods work. Men with testosterone that is normal for their age would have all the same forms of supplementation available to them—if their doctors agreed to let them try testosterone therapy.

If you wonder whether testosterone therapy might be right for you, talk with your doctor about the risks and benefits in your particular case. Treating normal aging with testosterone therapy is not generally recommended or considered advisable—but there are exceptions, and you may be one of them. But do *not* take testosterone supplements on your own: the ones sold on the Internet and through other non-prescription sources may not be effective and may be highly dangerous, containing too much or too little testosterone, or none

> *Treating normal aging with testosterone therapy is not generally recommended or considered advisable—but there are exceptions.*

at all—or additives that can themselves be dangerous. The fact that it is easy to obtain testosterone supplements does not mean that it is a good idea!

The Estrogen Issue

FOR WOMEN, testosterone issues take a back seat to ones involving the primary female sex hormone, *estrogen*. The body's diminishing production of estrogen near and at menopause is responsible for many symptoms with which women are all too familiar—and would rather not endure. Hot flashes are the most-often-discussed of these, but there are other important ones, including vaginal dryness, diminished sex drive, and reduced bone mass. These are female symptoms comparable to those caused by testosterone decrease in men—but women's symptoms are often more severe and rapid in onset, since menopause is a definite demarcation in a woman's life and there is nothing comparable to it in men.

Because women's menopausal symptoms can be severe, hormone replacement therapy—using medications containing female hormones to replace the ones the body no longer makes after menopause—used to be a standard treatment for women with hot flashes and other menopausal symptoms. Many women receiving the treatment, which usually combined estrogen with another hormone called *progesterone*, would certainly have described these as healing hormones. To make hormone therapy—as it is now called—even more attractive, it was thought to have major long-term benefits, including prevention of heart disease and possibly of dementia.

> Hormone replacement therapy used to be a standard treatment for women with hot flashes and other menopausal symptoms.

Risks Outweigh Benefits

BUT THEN a large clinical trial found that the treatment actually posed more health risks than benefits for many women—and the use of hormone therapy changed dramatically. Within a relatively short time, hormone therapy stopped being recommended for prevention of conditions such as heart disease or memory loss, and is no longer used as a disease preventative.

And then things got even more complicated, as new research and further reviews of clinical trials showed that estrogen *can* be a healing hormone for *some* women, depending on their risk factors. Long-term systemic hormone therapy for the prevention of

> Estrogen can be a healing hormone for some women.

postmenopausal conditions is no longer routinely recommended by doctors. But some data suggest that estrogen can decrease the risk of heart disease when taken early in postmenopausal years.

More significantly for many women, systemic estrogen—which is available in pill, skin patch, gel, cream or spray form—is still considered the most effective treatment for relief of menopausal hot flashes and night sweats. Estrogen can also ease vaginal symptoms of menopause, such as dryness, itching, burning and discomfort during intercourse. And the Food and Drug Administration still approves estrogen for the prevention of the bone-thinning disease called osteoporosis—although doctors now usually recommend medications called *bisphosphonates* to treat osteoporosis, rather than estrogen.

Fast-Changing Field

HORMONE THERAPY FOR WOMEN is a fast-changing field in which new research is constantly being conducted. But some things about hormone therapy are now accepted in the scientific and medical fields. In the largest clinical trial to date, a combination pill containing estrogen and progestin—a synthetic form of progesterone—increased the risk of serious conditions, including heart attack, stroke, blood clots and breast cancer. Women who took estrogen alone and had previously had a hysterectomy had higher risks of blood clots and strokes, but not breast cancer or heart disease.

These findings were enough to stop the routine use of hormone therapy for women in general. But the benefits may outweigh the risks for certain women, including those who are otherwise healthy but experience moderate to severe hot flashes or other menopausal symptoms; have lost bone mass and either cannot tolerate other treatments or are not benefiting from them; and those who had premature menopause—

> Low-dose vaginal hormonal products are generally considered safe.

meaning periods stopping before age 40—or premature ovarian insufficiency, meaning loss of normal ovarian function before age 40.

Furthermore, *low-dose* vaginal hormonal products *are* generally considered safe. They come in cream, tablet or ring form, and can effectively treat vaginal menopausal symptoms and some urinary symptoms. Absorption into the body is minimized, which is why women can generally use these products without worry—although it is still important to talk with your doctor about them. These locally applied preparations do not help with hot flashes, night sweats or osteoporosis protection.

The days have passed in which estrogen, alone or in combination, was deemed a healing hormone for women in general. But just as testosterone therapy can be of significant benefit for some men without being helpful to men in general, so hormone therapy with estrogen can be highly beneficial to some women under certain circumstances. Because knowledge in this field is so fluid, it is particularly necessary to discuss the pros and cons with your doctor.

14:

Human Growth Hormone

S UPPOSE YOU HAVE READ about testosterone and estrogen and come to realize that they are not panaceas for the slow decline of bodily functions that we call aging—and that testosterone and estrogen supplements are not helpful, and could be harmful, for people whose decline in the hormones is a natural part of the aging process rather than the effect of a disease. You may nevertheless find yourself wondering whether there is some *other* hormone that could keep the aging process at bay, and perhaps even reverse it. After all, the decline in levels of specific hormones *is* associated with a number of the effects of aging, including loss of bone density and muscle mass and an increase in body fat. Surely if there is a hormone associated with those aging-related declines, it should be possible to supplement the body's supply and reverse some of the effects of aging.

This line of thinking will likely lead you to one specific conclusion, because there *is* one particular hormone whose drop over time is strongly correlated with human aging. It is human growth hormone, HGH.

The Master Gland

HUMAN GROWTH HORMONE is produced by the pituitary gland, a structure at the base of the brain that is only the size of a pea and that weighs less than one-fifth of an ounce, but that has enormous importance in how humans grow, develop and age.

The pituitary secretes and stores hormones that control the functions of your body's other glands. It is a kind of control room for hormones and hormonal effects, and for that reason is sometimes called the master gland. The pituitary's hormones go on to control glands that in turn regulate such body functions as temperature, urine production, thyroid activity, and the production of sex hormones. Specifically, the pituitary produces eight different types of hormones—one of which is HGH.

It is because the pituitary gland acts as a master controller of other glands that its production of HGH lends credibility to the notion of HGH as a kind of anti-aging agent. Here is how this works. The pituitary receives messages from the *hypothalamus,* a part of the brain that gets information from the external environment and from other areas of your body. If one of your hormone levels drops too low, your hypothalamus sends a message—using the hormones it secretes—to your pituitary gland. In response,

> *The pituitary gland is a kind of control room for hormones and hormonal effects.*

your pituitary gland secretes hormones of its own and sends them through your bloodstream.

Hormones, remember, are chemical messengers, and the message they take from the pituitary to a misbehaving gland is to shape up and do its job better. If a gland has not been producing enough of its own hormones, the hypothalamus finds out, sends a message to the pituitary, and the pituitary sends a message to that gland to increase production of whatever hormones it makes. Similarly, if a gland is overproducing hormones, your pituitary gland sends it a message to lower its hormone production.

As We Age

AS WE GET OLDER, the pituitary becomes less efficient—and this is seen in particular in what happens with HGH production. The pituitary's HGH fuels childhood growth and helps maintain our tissues and organs throughout life. But starting in middle age, the pituitary gland slowly reduces the amount of growth hormone it produces. And as this happens, our tissues and organs begin to show signs of wear and deterioration. So it seems logical to ask whether *increasing* the amount of human growth hormone in our bodies will slow the decline of our bodies, slowing our physical progress into old age and helping us regain the youth and vitality we experienced when our levels of growth hormone were higher.

> H GH *can increase bone density and muscle mass, decrease body fat and boost exercise capacity.*

There is, in fact, good evidence that HGH can increase bone density and muscle mass, decrease body fat and boost exercise capacity. Synthetic human growth hormone, which must be injected and is available only by prescription, provides all those benefits to people with *growth hormone deficiency*. That is a rare condition generally caused by *pituitary adenoma*—a tumor on the pituitary gland—or by treatment of a pituitary adenoma with surgery or radiation. Synthetic HGH, which was developed in 1985 and is approved by the Food and Drug Administration for certain specific uses, is also effective in some people with muscle wasting related to AIDS or HIV.

When HGH Helps

HOWEVER, as with testosterone supplements, injected synthetic HGH has proven beneficial effects only when people have reduced levels of body-made HGH because of disease, not when lower HGH levels are simply attributable to the natural decline associated with aging. Also as with testosterone, studies of healthy adults taking human growth hormone are limited—and the ones that have been done have produced some unexpected, counterintuitive results. For example, although it appears that human growth hormone injections can increase muscle mass and reduce the amount of body fat in healthy older adults, the increase in muscle does not translate into increased strength.

Injected HGH also has a wide variety of side effects in healthy adults. It can cause carpal tunnel syndrome, arm and leg swelling, joint and muscle pain, and *gynecomastia* in men—that is, enlargement of breast tissue. It can cause the body's tissues to retain fluid, resulting in a condition called *edema*. And it can increase the risk of diabetes and heart disease.

Furthermore, research suggests that side effects of human growth hormone treatments may be more likely in older adults—the people most likely to want the supplements in order to counter our bodies' natural reduction in HGH over time—than in younger adults. Because the studies of healthy adults taking human growth hormone have been short-term ones, it is not clear whether the side effects would eventually dissipate—or would become worse.

HGH Pills

WHAT ABOUT PILLS instead of shots? Easy-to-take pills
are what most people considering HGH supplementation think about using. Oral HGH products—usually
pills and sometimes sprays—have attracted a particularly large following among bodybuilders and some other
athletes, who use them in combination with anabolic
steroids to try to boost muscle mass. Since HGH is
known to increase bone density and muscle mass,
decrease body fat and boost exercise capacity in people
with growth hormone insufficiency, the thinking goes,
it should provide the same benefits to people who do
not have that condition.

And some people, athletes or not, simply wonder,
why not try HGH? The chance of turning back your
biological clock can certainly make HGH supplements
seem worthwhile.

Some promoters sell what they describe as a pill
form of HGH and claim that it produces results similar
to those from the injected version of the drug. Sometimes these dietary supplements are called human
growth hormone releasers. Companies that market
these products on TV
infomercials or online
claim they turn back
your body's biologi-
cal clock, reducing fat,
building muscle, restor-
ing hair growth and color, strengthening the immune
system, normalizing blood sugar, increasing energy and
improving sex life, sleep quality, vision, and memory. Quite a list!

> There is no scientific evidence to support claims by promoters of HGH products.

Unfortunately for those hoping for an anti-aging pill, there is no scientific evidence to support claims that these products have the same effects as prescription HGH, which is always given by injection. In fact, they may have no effect at all, may have nothing to do with HGH, and may be dangerous. Some companies have been censured by government agencies for false claims and have had to shut down—although they have often sprung up again under different names. There is no way to know what is actually in these companies' products, since HGH may only be legally dispensed by prescription.

And there is an unfortunate scientific reality that none of the "HGH pill" firms ever addresses: taken orally, HGH is digested by the stomach before it can be absorbed into the body. Any medication or supplement that we take by mouth must survive our potent stomach-acid environment in order to get into the bloodstream. HGH does not: it is simply destroyed by the digestive process. So even if some form of HGH is contained within pills, it cannot make it into the body.

If you do want to slow the effects of aging—and who doesn't?—it is through healthful lifestyle choices, such as eating a good-for-you diet and including physical activity in your daily routine, that you can feel your best as you get older. Of course, this reality will not stop people from seeking an anti-aging pill: the search for the fountain of youth is many centuries old, and will likely go on indefinitely.

Hence the attraction of "HGH pills" and, for that matter, testosterone and estrogen supplements. It is natural to think that there *must* be healing hormones out there for the effects of aging! In fact, wouldn't it be great if there were a single hormone that would build our strength and sex drive *and* hold aging at bay? Some people think there is—as we will see in the next chapter.

15:

DHEA

YOU MAY RECALL that endorphins get their name from the words "endogenous morphine," referring to a body-produced morphine-like substance. Our bodies also produce *endogenous steroids*, and the single most abundant of these is *dehydroepiandrosterone,* known as DHEA. It is produced in the adrenal glands, which are located just above the kidneys, as well as in the gonads and in the brain—where it is important in our bodies' synthesis of androgen (male) and estrogen (female) sex hormones.

To understand the importance of DHEA, we need to look at some confusion and concern about steroids in general. Steroids have a mixed reputation, partly because of misuse of certain substances and partly because of misunderstanding. Scientifically, a steroid is simply a compound that has a characteristic chemical structure consisting of multiple rings of connected atoms. This means that estrogen is a steroid, and so is cholesterol, and so is vitamin A—even though we do not normally think of any of these substances when we hear the word "steroid."

> *Steroids have a mixed reputation, partly because of misuse and partly because of misunderstanding.*

Compounding the confusion is the word *corticosteroids*, which refers to a class of drugs used to treat arthritis and many other conditions. These drugs are often called *glucocorticoids* or simply referred to as "steroids," and that deepens the confusion. These drugs, which are potent anti-inflammatories but can have significant side effects, are not ones that anyone would consider using as supplements. But despite the similar name, the steroid DHEA is not the same as these medical steroids.

The Anabolics

AND THEN there are *anabolic* steroids, synthetic substances related to the male sex hormones, known as androgens. Anabolic steroids *are* used as supplements—and widely abused. They promote growth of skeletal muscle and the development of male sexual characteristics—and have often been used and misused by bodybuilders and other athletes seeking physical advantages over opponents.

Anabolic steroids are available legally only by prescription. They are used to treat conditions that occur when the body produces abnormally low amounts of testosterone, such as delayed puberty and some forms of impotence. They may also be prescribed to treat body wasting in AIDS and for use with other diseases that result in the loss of lean muscle mass.

Athletes' abuse of anabolic steroids is what has given steroids of all types a bad name, and it is certainly true that misuse of anabolic steroids has serious consequences. Anabolics can cause liver and kidney tumors, cancer, high blood pressure, jaundice, severe acne and trembling. In men, they can cause breasts to develop and testicles to shrink. In women, they can cause growth of facial hair, menstrual changes and deepening of voice.

Where DHEA Fits In

NONE OF THIS SOUNDS much like the fountain of youth! But as with medical corticosteroids, anabolic steroids are not the same thing as the steroid DHEA—and while supplementation with anabolics can be quite dangerous, supplementation with DHEA has a lot to recommend it. If we cut through the confusion and focus specifically on DHEA, we find a substance with some remarkable properties and having some claim to be a healing hormone—at least for some people and under some circumstances.

Like testosterone and HGH, DHEA—the most abundant steroid made by our bodies—is produced in greater amounts when we are young, and its levels gradually decrease in later life, beginning to drop after about age 30. DHEA levels are reported to be low in some people with anorexia, end-stage kidney disease, type 2 diabetes, AIDS, and adrenal insufficiency, and levels may also be reduced by a number of drugs, including insulin and opiates—and medical corticosteroids. Therefore, the thinking goes, higher levels of DHEA ought to help protect us against a variety of diseases and should slow the effects of aging itself.

In fact, a wide variety of claims have been made for supplementation of this hormone. It supposedly builds up the adrenal gland, strengthens the immune system, boosts energy, improves mood and memory, builds up muscle strength, and indeed—taking its effects as a whole—slows the natural bodily changes that come with age.

> Like testosterone and HGH, DHEA is produced in greater amounts when we are young.

Furthermore, DHEA is readily and legally available as a dietary supplement in the United States, being sold under such names as Fidelin and Ovomax. And it is specifically exempted from the Anabolic Steroid Control Act of 1990 and 2004, although it is banned from use in athletic competition. Other countries treat DHEA differently—for example, Canada and Australia require a prescription for it—but it tends to be reasonably easy to obtain. It also seems to be reasonably safe in short-term use: researchers have found few adverse short-term effects, although the long-term safety of DHEA supplementation is unknown, with studies reaching different conclusions.

DHEA's Value

WHAT CAN DHEA do for you? The answer is difficult to pin down, because scientists are not sure of everything that DHEA naturally does in the body. Because DHEA regulates the production and use of 18 other body-produced steroid hormones, including estrogen and testosterone, it is definitely vital to a variety of the body's systems. And because a slowdown in DHEA production is associated with various elements of aging, the thinking is that supplementation with DHEA may slow and reduce aging's toll on the body.

Things get tricky where DHEA is concerned, for the simple reason that it is not fully understood and research into it is ongoing. It is best to think of DHEA as a sort of "vitality hormone." DHEA seems to help relieve mild to moderate depression, and to be effective when used with regular treatment for obesity, systemic lupus and adrenal insufficiency. DHEA can cause higher than normal levels of androgen and estrogen in the body, and its proponents consider that a good thing, since raising those sex hormones can be seen as a sign of "reversing aging"—because production of the hormones normally declines with age. However, the heightened levels of androgen and estrogen may increase the risk of prostate, breast, ovarian, and other hormone-sensitive cancers—so simply boosting sex-hormone levels does not really improve health.

Proponents of DHEA say that using it regularly can have a significant impact on a wide variety of illnesses, especially ones associated with aging. They argue that taking it as a supplement can reduce the likelihood of heart disease, Alzheimer's, cervical cancer and Crohn's disease; that it can help prevent low bone density, head off chronic fatigue syndrome and protect against rheumatoid arthritis; that it fights psoriasis and schizophrenia; and that it protects against infertility and sexual dysfunction.

Miracle Hormone?

DHEA'S KNOWN INVOLVEMENT in the body's production of estrogen and testosterone makes claims for it involving sexual dysfunction and infertility reasonable. Some of the other claims, though, seem more like wish fulfillment than science—if they were all true, DHEA would be not just a healing hormone but a miracle hormone.

Unfortunately, the National Institutes of Health have found little evidence for DHEA's value in conditions such as Alzheimer's disease, rheumatoid arthritis, schizophrenia and other diseases. For example, a version of DHEA supplement known as 7-Keto has been widely promoted to help reduce body fat and raise metabolism—the idea being that leaner body tissue and higher metabolism will burn calories more efficiently, making it easier to lose weight and keep it off. Unfortunately, most scientific studies have shown that DHEA has little if any effect on weight loss or increased metabolism.

DHEA supplements have nevertheless been particularly popular with athletes because of claims that the substance can improve muscle strength and enhance athletic performance. DHEA is generally banned from athletic competitions because it can increase the body's levels of steroid hormones—such as testosterone. But there is little if any evidence that DHEA can enhance muscle strength, and it does carry significant risks when used in higher doses, as athletes have been known to do.

Negatives

ALTHOUGH THE POSITIVE EFFECTS of DHEA are not fully understood and are still being studied, with new information emerging regularly, the negative side effects—especially when DHEA is taken in higher doses—*are* known. They include permanent stunting of growth; aggressive behavior, sometimes referred to as "roid rage"; mood swings and other psychological symptoms; higher blood pressure; changes in cholesterol levels; liver problems; and sleep disturbances.

Despite these risks, DHEA supplementation is tempting for many of us. Short-term use, usually in an attempt to boost overall vitality, seems to have a low chance of troubling side effects. Some scientific studies—although by no means all—indicate that DHEA can help boost testosterone levels, and in fact it is used regularly to

> DHEA *does have importance to a wide variety of bodily processes.*

help treat female infertility. And even though DHEA's functions are not fully understood, given the fact that DHEA is the body's most abundant circulating steroid hormone, it clearly has importance to a wide variety of bodily processes. Many people believe it is reasonable to think that the overall slowing of the body that we know as aging is due in part to decreasing levels of DHEA— and if that is true, raising those levels ought to hold at least some signs of aging in check, even if they cannot be reversed.

Much Unknown

UNFORTUNATELY for those looking for certainty, all these thoughts are speculative, since there is much about DHEA that is still not known. And even if DHEA can slow some signs of aging in some people, it is a far cry from a hormonal fountain of youth. Further-more, some approaches to raising DHEA may sound logical but simply do not work. For example, DHEA can be synthesized in the lab using chemicals found in wild yam and soy. So some people eat soy to raise DHEA levels, and wild yam extract is sold in pill form by various companies as a "natural alternative" to syn-thetically produced DHEA supplements. This may be a good market niche—but the fact is that soy and wild yam cannot be converted into DHEA by the body, even though scientists can make the conversion in the lab by extraction of specific chemicals. As with so many ele-ments of our bodies' hormonal makeup, things are more complicated than they may at first seem to be.

In fact, since the claims and uncertainties surround-ing DHEA *are* so complicated, it is worth summarizing them. Proponents of DHEA supplementation say it can slow or reverse aging processes in general, and specifically can improve thinking skills in older people and slow the progress of Alzheimer's disease. It has been suggested as a way to prevent heart disease, breast cancer, diabetes, and metabolic syndrome, to boost the immune system in general, and to treat systemic *lupus erythematosus*, osteoporosis, multiple sclerosis, depression, schizophrenia, chronic fatigue syndrome, and Parkinson's disease. Some people say it eases depression and fatigue and can even help dieters lose weight.

Sexual Effects

THEN THERE ARE the supposed sexual effects of DHEA—which are supported by what scientists *do* know about its functions. It is sometimes used by men to treat erectile dysfunction; by healthy men and women who have low levels of certain hormones, to improve well-being and sexuality; to decrease the symptoms of menopause; and, in postmenopausal women, to strengthen the walls of the vagina and increase bone-mineral density.

And of course some athletes have been known to use DHEA to increase muscle mass, strength, and energy—although DHEA use is banned by athletic supervisory bodies.

There are so many varied claims for DHEA that it should be clear that a single substance—no matter how powerful—cannot possibly do everything it is claimed to do. And in fact, as we have seen, claims for most of these effects of DHEA are unsupported by scientific evidence; while for other claims, the evidence is mixed or insufficient to say for sure, one way or the other, whether DHEA is effective.

DHEA is known to have some effect in treating schizo-phrenia—apparently more in women than men. It can improve the appearance of older people's skin: taking DHEA by mouth seems to increase skin thickness and moisture, and decrease facial "age spots," in elderly men and women. It does seem to help some men with sexual dysfunction achieve an erec-tion—but not if their erec-tile dysfunction is caused by diabetes or nerve disorders.

> A single substance—no matter how power-ful—cannot possibly do everything that DHEA is claimed to do.

There is evidence that DHEA improves the symp-toms of lupus: taking DHEA by mouth along with con-ventional treatment seems to help reduce the number of times symptoms flare up, and may allow a reduction in the dose of prescription drugs needed. DHEA may also reduce lupus symptoms, such as muscle ache and mouth ulcers.

Helping Bones

DHEA ALSO HELPS people with weak bones, as seen in osteoporosis. Taking DHEA by mouth daily seems to improve bone mineral density in older women and men with osteoporosis or the pre-osteoporosis condition known as osteopenia. And it can boost bone-mineral density in young women with the eating disorder called anorexia nervosa.

This is an impressive list of effects, even if the "fountain of youth" claims for DHEA are overdone and unsupported. In fact, those claims—the ones that most people find exciting for DHEA—are either disproved by scientific evidence or simply not supported or de-nied, because there is not enough evidence one way or the other.

It is important to realize, in light of the many claims about DHEA, what this hormone does *not* do. There is no evidence that it fights Alzheimer's disease, improves the thinking abilities of healthy older people, or "reverses aging" in any meaningful way. It does not improve sexual arousal in healthy women, prevent breast cancer or heart disease, or cure chronic fatigue syndrome—although it may improve some symptoms of CFS in some patients. Similarly, DHEA does not reverse the course of HIV/AIDS, but may improve some patients' mental health and quality of life.

DHEA does not overcome metabolic syndrome, a cluster of conditions that puts people at high risk for heart disease. It might lower *some* of the health risks that make overweight men and women more likely to develop metabolic syndrome—including fat around the waist and high insulin levels. However, it does not promote weight loss for most people—although it does seem to help overweight older people who are likely to get metabolic syndrome lose weight.

And DHEA does not boost physical performance— some research shows that older adults who take DHEA have improved measures of muscle strength, but other research has found no effect on muscle strength of taking DHEA.

Much Unknown

IF THE PLUSES AND MINUSES of DHEA seem confusing, that is because this is a hormone that has so far resisted all attempts to pin down what it does and does not do. Therefore, considering DHEA supplementation requires thinking about *why* you may want to take it and deciding whether its known and unknown effects are in line with what you hope it will do for you.

If you decide that the known and potential benefits of DHEA make it worthwhile for you to try for a few months—DHEA is generally considered safe when taken for that amount of time—you should still talk to your doctor first. The fact that DHEA supplements are available without prescription in the United States can lend us a false sense of security about their safety. But DHEA is, after all, a hormone, and the whole point of hormone supplementation is to increase some things that the body does and/or decrease others.

The power of any hormone is both the reason to use it and the reason to be cautious about it. As an example, here is just one complication: DHEA can decrease the time the liver needs to break down some medications—and this can increase the effects and side effects of those medicines. These are not obscure drugs: they include lovastatin, sold as Mevacor®; ketoconazole, sold as Nizoral®; fexofenadine, sold as Allegra®; triazolam, sold as Halcion®; and many more. So, again, your doctor must know if you plan to take DHEA, and you yourself must be on the alert for any changes in your reaction to prescription medicines that you are taking at the same time as DHEA.

It would be stretching things to call DHEA a healing hormone in the way that nitric oxide, dopamine, endorphins, serotonin and oxytocin are. DHEA does not counter the stress response, as healing hormones do, and its effects are complex, not fully understood, and not supportive of the main reason so many of us would like to use it—to reverse the inevitable decline of an aging body. Still,

> The fact that DHEA supplements are available without prescription can lend us a false sense of security.

DHEA supplementation can have a positive impact on some conditions, as noted above, and using DHEA supplements in moderation, with your doctor's knowledge and agreement, and for a relatively short time, may boost your overall health and sense of well-being.

Complex Chemicals

HEALING HORMONES are complex chemicals whose effects are many and varied, and our body's elegantly balanced physical properties make it difficult for us to increase or decrease the levels of particular hormones for specific purposes without the risk of throwing our physical balance off in some other way. This is why inducing our bodies to make more of desirable hormones is better for our health than taking hormonal supplements, even when—as is the case with DHEA—such supplements are readily available.

The fact is that two hormone-boosting behaviors associated with the healing hormones will also raise DHEA naturally: exercise and a healthful, calorie-restricted diet. If you eat well and get regular physical activity, levels of both DHEA and the healing hormones will rise in your body naturally. Think of it as the body repaying you for taking better care of yourself. It may seem simpler to take a supplement than to change your living habits if you are not already eating healthfully and exercising regularly. But in the long run—and the long run is what all of us hope to be around for—encouraging your body to make more of its desirable

> Two hormone-boosting behaviors associated with the healing hormones will also raise DHEA naturally: exercise and a healthful, calorie-restricted diet.

hormones is a far better approach than looking for
shortcuts to boost one specific hormone or another. If
you treat your body well, it will respond by treating your
consciousness well—your mind, your soul, your spirit,
whatever you choose to call it. And that will give you
a life that is happier, healthier, and more hormonally
satisfying.

16:

Healing Hormones

THERE'S A LOT TO LEARN about our bodies' hormones, their effects and how you can get your body to make more of the substances that will make you feel better! Now that you have learned about what your body produces and how your behavior can affect your hormones and therefore your mood and overall feeling of well-being, here is an overview, hormone by hormone, that you can use to guide yourself in taking charge of your body and improving your own health.

Hormone	Effects	How to Boost
Nitric Oxide	Widens blood vessels, improves blood flow; prevents oxygen starvation; improves heart health; prevents strokes and heart attacks; fights infection; improves sexual response.	Increase arginine intake by eating more vegetables and nuts, garlic, onion, cold-water fish, eggs, chicken, green tea; exercise to get your heart beating faster.

Dopamine	Affects movement, emotions, memory, experience of pleasure; fights depression; boosts motivation; provides emotional balance.	Get more tyrosine from protein-rich foods and such fruits and vegetables as bananas and avocados, plus dairy products; exercise at least 20-30 minutes/day; have more sex; avoid foods high in cholesterol and added sugar; consider supplements of vitamins A, B6, C and E.
Endorphins	Create calm; relieve pain; encourage dopamine production.	Laugh or anticipate laughing; exercise at enough intensity to produce "runner's high"; massage therapy; acupuncture; inhale odors of vanilla and lavender; eat ginseng.

Serotonin	Relaxation and contentment; "happy hormone"; restful sleep; feelings of being at peace with the environment; protects against depression; improves social life.	Consume tryptophan-rich foods such as seafood, turkey, chicken, milk, eggs, nuts and other protein sources.
Oxytocin	Sexual bonding; pair attachment; mother-child connection; feelings of calm and security; promotes in-group attachment at the expense of out-group; boosts sensitivity to positive social cues.	Be affectionate with your partner in public and private; touch frequently; increase sexual foreplay; think pleasant thoughts; interact with a pet, especially through touch.

Testerostone (men)	Maintains bone density; manages fat distribution; maintains muscle strength & mass; affects red-blood-cell production; promotes sex drive & sperm production.	Supplements available as injections, pellets, patches or gels, but generally not recommended for men whose levels are normal for their age.
Estrogen (women)	Can relieve symptoms of menopause, decrease some women's heart-disease risk, help prevent osteoporosis.	Systemic supplements available as pills, skin patches, gels, creams or sprays. Long-term use not recommended & must be carefully supervised. Low-dose vaginal products are generally safe & effective for vaginal menopausal symptoms and some urinary symptoms—available as creams, tablets or rings.

Human Growth Hormone	Increases bone density and muscle mass, decreases body fat, boosts exercise capacity—but only in people with a deficiency.	Injections available only by prescription and must be medically administered. Claims for supposed pill form not supported by science.
DHEA	Regulates production of testosterone, estrogen & other hormones; helps relieve depression, treat schizophrenia, improves aging skin, may relieve lupus symptoms, improves bone density. Effects not fully known. May increase effects and side effects of many medicines.	Eat a healthful diet and exercise regularly. Available as a nutritional supplement, without a prescription, in the United States. So-called natural alternatives to synthetic DHEA—such as soy and wild yam—is not effective.

IMPORTANT: Even when hormone supplements are available without a prescription, that does not mean they are safe for everyone under all circumstances. Always discuss it with your doctor before taking any hormone supplement.

Bibliography

Alexander, Tyson, "Benefit of Endorphins," *Livestrong. com*, Jan. 20, 2011.

Bailey, Joshua, "What Are the Benefits of Nitric Oxide Supplements?" *Livestrong.com*, Mar. 14, 2011.

Benson, Herbert, *Beyond the Relaxation Response*. New York: Berkley, 1985.

Benson, Herbert, and Miriam Z. Klipper, *The Relaxation Response*. New York: HarperTorch, 2000.

Bergland, Christopher, "Let's Not Get Panicky: A Drug-Free Prescriptive to Reduce Stress," *Psychology Today*, Jan. 9, 2012.

Berk, Lee S., and Stanley A. Tan, "[beta]-Endorphin and HGH Increase are associated with both the anticipation and experience of mirthful laughter," *The FASEB Journal*, Mar. 2006,

Bezaitis, Athan, "How Nitric Oxide Maintains Health," *USC News*, Feb. 18, 2009.

Block, Will, "I'm in the Mood for Love...'simply' because of higher nerve growth factor levels," *Life Enhancement*, Nov. 2012,

DeAngeles, Tori, "Can Oxytocin Promote Trust and Generosity?" *American Psychological Association*, Vol. 39, No. 2, Feb 2008.

DeAngelis, Tori, "The Two Faces of Oxytocin," *American Psychological Association*, Vol. 39, No. 2, Feb. 2008.

De Dreu, Carsten K.W., Lindred L. Greer, Michel J.J. Handgraaf, et al., "The Neuropeptide Oxytocin Regulates Parochial Altruism in Intergroup Conflicts Among Humans," *Science*, Vol. 328, No. 5894, Jun. 11, 2010.

Grant, Nina, Mark Hamer and Andrew Steptoe, "Social Isolation and Stress-related Cardiovascular, Lipid, and Cortisol Responses," *Annals of Behavioral Medicine*, Feb. 5, 2009.

Hendrickson, Kirstin, "What Are the Benefits of Serotonin?" *Livestrong.com*, Sep. 2, 2010.

Hurlemann, René, Alexandra Patin, Oezguer A. Onur, et al., "Oxytocin Enhances Amygdala-Dependent, Socially Reinforced Learning and Emotional Empathy in Humans," *Journal of Neuroscience*, 5538-09, Apr. 7, 2010,

King, Joe, "Vitamins that Enhance Dopamine," *Livestrong.com*, May 8, 2011.

MacDonald, Ann, "Using the Relaxation Response to Reduce Stress," *Harvard Health Blog*, Nov. 10, 2010.

McDonald, Christina, "Dopamine Benefits," *Livestrong. com*, Dec. 19, 2009

Nelson, Roxanne, "Job Stress Doesn't Seem to Raise Risk for Cancer," *Medscape Medical News*, Feb. 8, 2013.

"9 Ways to Balance Your Hormones Naturally," *Global Healing Center*, May 1, 2011/Jun. 10, 2013.

"Nitric Oxide: Do You Have Enough of this Gas for Optimal Performance?" *NaturalHealthSherpa.com*, Apr. 16, 2012.

O'Connor, Kieran, "What Supplement Produces Dopamine in Your Brain?" *Livestrong.com*, Mar. 31, 2011

Scheele, Dirk, Nadine Striepens, Inur Güntürkün et al., "Oxytocin Modulates Social Distance Between Males and Females," *Journal of Neuroscience*, 2755-12, Nov. 14, 2012.

Scheiderer, Dave, "The Benefits of Natural Dopamine Supplements," *Integrative Psychiatry*, Apr. 27, 2010,

Sifferlin, Alexandra, "How a Healthy Heart Can Lower Risk of Cancer," *Time: Health & Family*, Mar. 19, 2013.

"Social Isolation Tied to Shorter Lifespan," *Medical News Today*, Mar. 27, 2013.

Steptoe, Andrew, Apama Shankar, Panayotes Demakakos and Jane Wardle, "Social isolation, loneliness, and all-cause mortality in older men and women," *Proceedings of the National Academy of Sciences*, Feb. 15, 2013.

Stoppler, Melissa Conrad, MD, "Endorphins: Natural Pain and Stress Fighters," MedicineNet.com. Mar. 15, 2007.

Szalavitz, Maya, "How a Squirt of Oxytocin Could Ease Marital Spats and Boost Social Sensitivity," *Time: Health & Family*, Aug. 14, 2012,

Szalavitz, Maia, "Social Isolation, Not Just Feeling Lonely, May Shorten Lives," *Time: Health & Family*, Mar. 26, 2013,

Szalavitz, Maia, "Stand By Your Man: Physical Proximity May Help Oxytocin to Keep Men in Relationships Faithful," *Time: Health & Family*, Nov. 14, 2012,

Wade, Nicholas, "Depth of the Kindness Hormone Appears to Know Some Bounds," *The New York Times*, Jan. 10, 2011,

Index

T

V

W

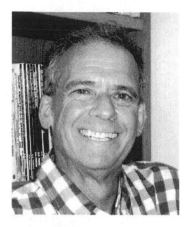

Mark J. Estren, Ph.D., received his doctorates in psychology and English from the University at Buffalo and his master's in journalism from Columbia University. He has written extensively on medical and health issues, specializing in communicating complex scientific information in easy-to-understand language and in explaining the implications for everyday life of cutting-edge research. A Pulitzer-winning journalist, he has held top-level positions at numerous news organizations for more than 30 years, including producer of "Report on Medicine" for CBS Radio, health-related reporting for the *Bottom Line Newsletters*, *The Washington Post*, *Miami Herald*, *Philadelphia Inquirer*, United Press International, and CBS and ABC News. His offices are in Fort Myers, Florida. (www.markjestren.com)

Beverly A. Potter, Ph.D, (Docpotter) received her doctorate in counseling psychology from Stanford University and her masters in vocational rehabilitation counseling from SFSU. She has authored numerous self-help books. Her offices are in Oakland, California. (www.docpotter.com)

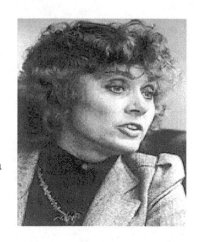

RONIN BOOKS FOR INDEPENDENT MINDS